Dedication

To my family; especially to my sister, Francine;
daughter Susanne; my son John;
aunt Yolanda and uncle Dave Carriero
who gave me love, advice,
support and encouragement.

Acknowledgements

I would like to give special thanks to Ron Davidson
who inspired the idea for, *So You Want To Be A Nurse*,
and who gave me exceptional help, advice and support
in making this book possible.

To my friends, Virgina and Verity Bostick;
Debbie Collins; Kathleen Conway-Gervais;
Ann Davidson, Lisa Hantverk, Theresa Munz,
Linda Murtagh, Julie Musiker, Mary Ann Pepe,
Susan Stern who gave me loving friendship,
encouragement and assistance.

To all the nurses who helped make this book
possible especially Chrissy Hudak, Doris Manna,
Debbie Musiker, Cindy Pigno, and Ann West.

TABLE OF CONTENTS

Scope, Plan and Purpose

So you Want to Be a Nurse? is a book for anyone who is or who ever wanted to be a nurse. The book reveals everything nobody else wants to tell you about the nursing profession. It shows how to save the reader the agony of on the job trial and error training and will give you a head start in using experienced strategies while dealing with administrators, physicians, technicians, colleagues, patients and their families. It is not about nursing techniques; it is about how to survive in a hospital once you get a nursing position. There are The Ten Commandments of Nursing, which sums up in ten steps how to survive in nursing and gives in-depth reasons why they work.

It is a refreshingly new and realistic book that touches on the reality that nurses may or may not succeed at nursing because of administrators, physicians, managers, colleagues, patients and their families and not because of their medical knowledge and expertise. It is a self-help book designed to successfully ease you into any nursing situation.

The chapter topics are:

Getting a Nursing Position
Salaries and Positions
Schooling, polices and procedures
Administrators, physicians, charge nurses and managers
Meet the Nurses
Patients and their families
Meetings
Patients and How to Protect yourself
Complaining
The Ten Commandments of Nursing.

Each of these topics will be discussed fully with real-life stories and examples. There will be easy steps given on how to handle each issue and how a nurse can ease into a hospital. The Ten Commandments will make it easy for you to sum up the do's and don'ts in order to survive in the nursing profession.

Preface

So You Want To Be A Nurse? conveys a realistic way of looking at a nurse's role. It tells you what no one else will tell you about nursing. Entertaining narrative stories are incorporated into the text to give the reader examples of real life nursing situations. These authentic tales show how nurses behave and react to each other, their supervisor, doctors, patients and their families, and how one can best handle each situation. The Ten Commandments of Nursing is provided as a guide to success in easing into any nursing situation. There is also a summary of the main ideas from the book presented in easy to remember fashion.

Anyone interested in nursing and the roles they play will find this book worthwhile reading. It is for anyone who wants to be a nurse, who is a nurse, has just started their career as a nurse, or college nursing majors. Anyone who is considering becoming a nurse or contemplating a change of careers will also find the facts as expressed in, *So You Want To Be A Nurse?* very influential in their decision-making. This book will provide you with a new outlook on life in the nursing field.

Introduction

So you Want to Be a Nurse? The book reveals everything nobody else wants to tell you about the nursing profession. It shows how to save the reader the agony of on the job trial and error training and will give you a head start in using experienced strategies while dealing with administrators, physicians, technicians, colleagues, patients and their families. It is not about nursing techniques; it is about how to survive in a hospital once you get a nursing position. There are The Ten Commandments of Nursing, which sums up in ten steps how to survive in nursing and gives in-depth reasons why they work.

It is a refreshingly new and realistic book that touches on the reality that nurses may not succeed at nursing because of administrators, physicians, technicians, colleagues, patients and their families and not because they don't know medical procedures. It is a self-help book designed to successfully ease you into any nursing situation.

The chapter topics are:

Getting a Nursing Position
Salaries and Positions
Schooling, policies and procedures
Administrators, physicians, charge nurses and managers
Meet the Nurses
Patients and their families
Meetings
Patients and How to Protect yourself
Complaining
The Ten Commandments of Nursing.

Each of these topics will be discussed fully with real-life stories and examples. There are easy steps given on how to handle each issue and how a nurse can ease into a hospital. The Ten Commandments makes it easy for you to sum up the dos and don'ts in order to survive in the nursing profession.

Chapter 1: Getting a Nursing Position
Why do you want to be a nurse?
How to find a nursing position
Which position might be best for you
Which institutions and salary level are right for you

In this chapter you will explore the reasons people go into nursing. Questions will be presented that will help you decide if and why you want to go into nursing. It gives realistic views on the issues of nursing, getting the right position, and what positions are available and where. Insights into what nursing is really like and what position will be best for you will be discussed. Different types of health facilities and nursing positions are reviewed. You will be able to decide which would be best for you. It also gives helpful hints on how to survive once you get a position.

Chapter 2: Salaries and Positions
Different nursing positions salaries
Typical nursing positions
Careers outside traditional nursing setting

This chapter will introduce you to the different nursing positions and their duties. It will help you know what is the right position for you and what you can expect in salaries and duties. Untraditional nursing position are also discussed which will give you new and exciting prospective about nursing. This chapter will give you some usual as well as unusual vocations in nursing while giving you some idea of salary and training. After reading this chapter you will have a better idea of what position would be right for you.

Chapter 3: Schooling, Policies and Procedures
Educational requirements for every type of nursing
Polices and procedures of the nursing profession
American Nurses Association and National League of Nursing
History of nursing

This chapter explains what type of schooling you will need for whatever type of nurse you choose to be. You will also learn the different polices and procedures of the nursing profession in order to succeed. This chapter will show you how a hospital is a business and how to succeed in it. It gives you insights into the beginnings of the American Nurses Association and the National League of Nursing. Their rules, regulations, and general beliefs will be discussed. It tells when the union has power and when it doesn't. This chapter will show you how to find the place to work for that has the least amount of conflicting issues.

Other concerns will also be dealt with in this chapter, such as: What can the union really do for me? Who is really going to fight for me if I have a problem with a supervisor, patient or co-worker? How will working in certain positions and facilities help my chances of easing into a new position?

Chapter 4: Administrators, Physicians, Charge Nurses and other managers
       Fair charge nurse
       How to collaborate with coworkers
       Physician-nurse relationship
       Relationships with nursing supervisors
       How to make the favorites and supervisors like you
       How to find a fair supervisor
       What affects your evaluation
       Building a support group

This chapter tells you how and why you must find a fair charge nurse to work under. New nurses usually are assigned to a unit and don't get to choose their charge nurse but there are things you can do to find a fair charge nurse and this chapter explains them. It also explains how to get the charge nurse to like you. It will acquaint you with the social structure you will encounter at any institution where you will be working. It will awaken you to the pecking order and how to succeed in it. The powers of the administrators/board of trustees, department heads, physicians, nursing service director, charge nurse, registered nurse, nurse practitioners, nurses aids, patients and families will be discussed and how they can effect your nursing position.

It will answer questions such as: To whom other then the charge nurse and nurse supervisor do I listen? How can I get a good evaluation and when and how do I get to know the higher-ups? How can I avoid being the victim of the higher pecking order? How do I build a support group? It also gives helpful rules on how to interact with your fellow workers for successful acceptance.

Chapter 5: Meet the Nurses

> Personalities of nurses
> Something special to offer nurse, the mother figure nurse, ethical value nurse, personal integrity nurse, military nurse, and inner city school nurse,
> Nursing and substance abuse

This chapter shows you the typical nurse personalities and how to learn from them. It will show you what type of personalities you will encounter when you enter a health facility. Examples from the almost –perfect nurse to the most imperfect nurse are depicted. It will give you insights into what you should model your personality from in order to succeed.

There are many types of nurses described. Margaret the nurse who can work with the terminally ill patient, Mindy the soft spoken compassionate nurse who helps her patients get in touch with their feelings, Marie the extremely religious nurse who believes in preserving life at all cost even if it means going against the patient and family wishes, and Joe the liberal male nurse who doesn't judge people. From these personalities you will learn how to avoid the traps they fell into and how to protect yourself. They will enlighten you in your own beliefs and how to deal with them to succeed in nursing.

Chapter 6: Patients and Their Families

> How to establishing a constructive relationship with patients and their families

How to handle families that can't cope, families who keep information from the patient, and families that blame themselves.

What to do if the family solution is in conflict with the patient's

When to speak up for your patient

In this chapter the hard facts are given about what a nurse has control over when dealing with patients and their families. Realistic suggestions touching upon how to deal with patient and families when faced with difficult situations for achieving best results are discussed. Interesting anecdotes will show the best answers to difficult patient problems, and case studies are given about difficult patient and families and which strategies lead to success in dealing with them.

Many questions are discussed in this chapter, such as: What do you do when the family keeps information from the patient? Are you supposed to take sides if the family's solution is in conflict with the patient's? How do you help the family that can't cope?

Helpful hints on how to talk to a family to get best results are also given. This chapter will provide you with helpful hints for successfully dealing with any family patient situation.

Chapter 7: Meetings

Different meetings and what each accomplishes

How to behave at meetings

How to interview a patient

What information to give to a patient

This chapter will give you information in order to make meetings work for you. Many different types of meetings are discussed such as staff meetings, family/patient meetings and how to interview a patient. Suggestion will be given on how to conduct yourself for best results and helpful hints will be provided. Sample meetings are depicted which give you a good picture of what to expect at any meeting. Helpful hints on how to conduct a patient interview for best results are given. When and what information to give a patient is discussed. Sample interviews are provided with hints for getting the most out of your interviews. With the helpful hints provided in this chapter you will be able to make any type of meeting work for you.

Chapter 8: Patients and How to Protect Yourself
Physical and mentally caring for your patients
How to handle the angry, guilty, in denial, fearful, and depressed patients
Spiritual issues
Dealing with death of a patient
Laws and your rights
When to listen and what to tell a patient
How to protect yourself emotionally

In this chapter the hard facts are given about what a nurse has control over when he or she is confronted with difficult patients. It also deals with how a nurse has to care for the patient's physical as well as mental health. Different personalities of patient's are discussed and suggestions are given on how to best solve the problems associated with each personality. Questions are answered on how to help an angry patient direct his anger in a positive way. Also how to help a guilt ridden patient cope, how to help a patient in denial realize, accept and find solution to his illness, how to help a fearful patient put his fear in proper prospective, and know when a depressed patient needs professional help.

In this chapter, your rights and the law will be reviewed. It will tell you when to listen to a patient and how much to tell them. It will give you helpful hints on how to emotionally protect yourself. This chapter also discusses spiritual issues and how to best deal with them in a neutral way. Helpful hints are given on how to cope with a patient's death to insure your healthy mental state.

Chapter 9: Complaining

How to constructively complain
Doctor and nurses relationships
Healthy nurses relationships
How to be optimistic
When and how to say "No"

This chapter shows what a nurse can do to learn how to complain constructively. Constructive complaining is when you know who to complain to and how you can do it to reap the most positive results. This chapter will explain the steps to learn successful constructive complaining. You will learn in what situations you should complain and how to complain effectively.

Doctors and nurses relationships are discussed. Question like" Why can't I argue with a doctor? Why can't I tell him he is wrong? Helpful hints on how to achieve a healthy and rewarding relationship with your fellow nurses are given. Optimistic verses pessimistic point of view are reviewed and shown how they can affect your success as a nurse. Ideas on how to achieve and keep an optimistic point of view are given. After you have read this chapter you will have a better understanding on when and how to complain to succeed in the nursing profession.

Chapter 10: The Ten Commandments of Nursing

The Ten Commandments of Nursing
1. Find the right environment for your professional goals
2. Interact cooperatively with physicians
3. Follow policies, procedures and nursing standards
4. Don't alienate your co-workers
5. Don't put your own beliefs ahead of the patient's
6. Don't alienate the patient's family
7. Choose your work friends cautiously
8. Complain Constructively
9. Don't Monopolize Meetings
10. Do extras for the supervisors

This chapter gives details on how to fulfill the Ten Commandments of Nursing in order to achieve a successful entry into any health facility. The entertaining and interesting stories from the book will be reviewed for solutions to any problems with administrators, physicians, colleagues, patients and their families to make your nursing career easier, thus finding an easy entry into any nursing position.

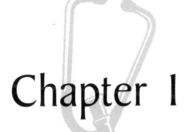

Chapter 1

Getting a Nursing Position

There can be many reasons why you would want to be a nurse. You should ask yourself many questions before you decide to become a nurse. Why do you want to be a nurse? What reasons do you give yourself for wanting to go into nursing? What are the positive reasons for wanting to go into nursing? Is it gratification or power? Is it the gratification of helping others? Is it power of healing? Why do you want to spend so much time with sick people? Have you been around and taken care of sick people? What do you want from your patients and their families? Do you feel compassion for people? What can you give them? Do you want them to listen to everything you say in their healing process? Will you be able to be firm but empathetic? How much do you need them to like you? Will you be afraid to persuade them to abide by medical procedures? What kind of patients do you expect to work with? Will you be able to work with patients different from what you expect? Will you be able to work in a hospital that does not meet your expectations?

Nurses have been portrayed as saints and sex objects, women both dedicated and servile, treasured but not necessarily respected. Today, even the positive depictions of nurses leave the impression that their work, along with their intelligence, is secondary to that of the doctors. Nurses prevent bad things from happening and it's much more difficult to measure what doesn't happen as opposed to what does. Some people believe a nurse needs a strong back, weak mind and little else. They feel people become nurses because they never considered the possibilities of other medical roles. Young people today are sometimes discouraged by their high school counselors and families from being "just a nurse." When you get into the profession you will realize that nursing requires a strong back, a keen mind and a very strong will. You should become aware of your own motivation before becoming a nurse and make your own judgments about the nursing profession.

The definition of nursing is a combination of the art of caring and the science of healthcare. Those in the nursing professions are concerned with particular health problems, but they also focus on patients and how they respond to treatment. Registered nurses (RN's) are people who work to promote health, prevent disease, and help patients deal with and heal from illness. They are advocates and health educators for patients, families, and communities. They provide direct patient care by assisting physicians, administering medication, and tending to patients' convalescence and reha-bilitation. They also observe, assess and record symptoms, reactions, and progress. RN's develop and manage nursing care plans; instruct patients and their families in proper care; and help individual and groups to take steps to maintain and improve their health. The work setting usually deter-mines their day to day job duties.

Now why do you want to be a nurse? You should become aware of your own motivations before becoming a nurse. Is it for the love of help-ing people? Is it because you want to work with people and value the rewards nursing has to offer? Most nurses have a need and desire to work with people. Do you fall into this category?

Another reason people find nursing rewarding is the knowledge of healing. They find trying to understand the healing process fascinating.

They like the idea of healing people and seeing the process in action. Some people say as long as they can remember they wanted to be a nurse. They can always remember wanting to take care of people and trying to make them well.

When most of us think of nurses, we call to mind helpful caring people. Maybe you remember a nurse who calmed you down and made you feel secure and took care of you. We may also think of nurses who taught us how to stay healthy and gave us good medical advice in time of need.

Many reasons lead people into nursing. Some people go into nursing because they like helping sick people and watching them get better. Some feel they accomplish something for their patients when they see them get well. Nursing can be a rewarding experience, which some people need and want. Nursing may be a way of using the power of persuading people to value and deepen their health beliefs.

Decide If You Want To Be a Nurse

Choosing to become a nurse is not a light decision. Some issues you may want to examine to help in the decision-making are:
Examine your motives for becoming a nurse. What is motivating you to become a nurse? Can you develop positive personality traits that will help in nursing? Do you have or can you develop personality traits that you feel a nurse should have? Will you be able to learn a variety of approaches to patient care? Are you interested in medical procedure and trying different medical techniques? Can you embrace unfamiliar communities and cultures and work with them? Do you want to work in unfamiliar communities and cultures? Can you understand different cultures? Can you fulfill the needs of your patients? Are you able to not use your own belief and instead comply with the patient's wishes.Will you be able to handle the procedures of the job and also deal with verbal and physical conflict? Will you be able to handle all types of patients? Will you be able to understand and accept the social structure and politics of the hospital or institution where you work? Will you be able to meet the specific needs of any patient? Will you have an awareness of the communities and the people in

dealing with any type of conflict? Can you learn to accept criticism and be humble?

Knowing what you want to do and why is the first step in finding personal and professional satisfaction. Few of us ever take the opportunity to think about what we want or how much control we have in achieving these goals. Take a few minutes now to commit your goals on paper. Separate a sheet of paper into two columns. At the top of the left side, write "Personal Goals," and on the top of the right, write "Professional Goals." On the first side, begin each statement with: ***Whom I want in my life: What I want in my life: Where I want to be in my life: When I will get these in my life and How I will get these in my life.*** Then complete your statements as specifically as you can. On the second side of the paper, begin each statement with, "As a nurse, whom would I want in my life," etc. Write the answers to these statements. These lists may give you some idea of where you want to be in a few years from now. When you have finished, look at the two lists. Are some of your professional goals the same as your personal goals? Will nursing help you to attain some of your personal goals? For example on your personal goal list you may have written, "I want to be with family and friends I can love and help," and on your professional goal list you may have written, "As a nurse I want to be helpful and take care of people." From this comparison you should be able to see that your professional goals and your personal goals are somewhat harmonious. Through nursing you are able to reach toward some of your personal goals. If you find that they do not coincide at all, you may want to reevaluate either your personal or professional goals.

What It Is Like To Be A Nurse

Nursing is not sitting a bedside vigil by candlelight, bathing damp brows, nor is it cracking open a chest every five minutes like you see on "ER". Nursing is rarely glamorous, and it is hard work but it is also deeply rewarding. On a daily basis, a nurse is a caregiver, counselor, teacher, client advocate, collaborator and critical thinker. Nurses blend science and art to achieve healing, health maintenance and health promotion. There are no "typical" days because the profession is so diverse.

Nursing can be a very rewarding profession, It can also be very stressful and challenging. Nurses must be able to communicate not only with patients, but also with physicians, administrators, and technicians. Their work often goes unnoticed or taken for granted. The problem and unknowns of nursing should not be overly stressed. In some ways nursing comes naturally to people who are nurturing caring individuals who get great satisfaction out of caring for sick or injured people.

While every nurse brings unique personal qualities to the profession, there are some common denominators among the really great ones. Some ideas that will help you become an effective nurse are:

The well being of the patient is the first priority.
Take time to reassure worried patients and boost morale.
Learn to recognize and understand patients' emotional as well as physical needs.
Know when to alert doctors or charge nurses about a patient's condition.
Be receptive to the families' request.
Have empathy and tolerance
Have strong organizational skills
Have well developed critical thinking skills
Have excellent communication skills
Have affinity for life long learning , teaching and caring for clients

How To Find A Nursing Position

The job opportunities for nurses are very optimistic. There are many opportunities in the health profession for nursing positions. The fastest growing professional opportunities are concentrated in the health-care services, which are expected to increase more than twice as fast as other sectors of the economy. The increased demand for healthcare services is expected to continue for a full 50 years. This is especially true right now as the Baby Boomers are becoming seniors. There is a good chance of finding a nursing position. You may not at first get the shift you desire but you should be able to get the position you desire.

Registered nurses' employment is expected to grow faster than the average for all healthcare occupations. There will be a need for traditional hospital nurses, but a large number of new nurses will be employed in home health, long term, nursing homes, community services and ambulatory care.

Most nurses work in hospitals taking care of sick people and helping them. Nurses also work in other places. Visiting nurses go to the homes of the sick. Some nurses assist in the offices of doctors and dentists. Others work in medical clinics, in schools, in retail businesses and industry, in the armed forces, and on ships, trains, and airplanes.

Nurses also help healthy people stay well. They teach children and adults to protect themselves from disease. Nurses who have had an advanced education may also teach in schools and colleges of nursing.

The two main groups of nurses are professional nurses and technical nurses. Professional nurses are usually graduates of four or five year college programs. Technical nurses are graduates of two-year community college or three-year hospital programs. Another group of nurses is called practical nurses. They need to complete a training program that generally last 12 months. They perform many duties that free up time for the professional and technical nurses to handle tasks that requires more specialized knowledge and experience.

While the private hospital industry is expected to grow slowly, employment in offices of health practitioners and in nursing and personal care facilities is expected to grow faster than in most other sectors. Healthcare manpower shortages are now commonplace and many healthcare providers take months to locate qualified personnel.

Knowing the normal salary range in your profession and in your location can be important in deciding which job offer to accept. Salaries for Registered Nurses can vary greatly depending on the geographic location and specific job setting as well as the education and experience of the individual. According to a 2002 National League for Nurses (NLN) RN's working full time have an earning ranging from $34,000 to $95,000 or more. Median annual salary for a registered nurse is $43,000. Median annual earning in industries employing the largest numbers of registered nurses are; Personnel supply services $48,000, Hospitals $44,000. Nursing and personal care facilities $39,000. Many employers offer flexible work schedules, childcare, educational benefits, and bonuses.

You will probably have no trouble getting a staff nursing position. For other types of positions such as supervisors or managerial positions you may need to do a little more work. The surest way to get a position is to know someone, preferably a supervisor who is in charge of hiring or who knows someone who is. If you don't know any supervisors through family of friends, then you should network. Join a nursing organization that has supervisors as members with whom you can congregate. Going through connections is the best way to get a good position. After that individuals must identify viable employment opportunities through associations, newsletters, Internet sites, directories, job fairs, personal contacts, job hotlines, corporations, placement agencies, and other published listings.

When researching places of employment you not only need to decide where you would fit in the best, but also which institution would be best for you. Decide what the three most important things you want from an employer and find out which employer will give them to you. Maybe money is one of your most important criteria for accepting a position. Or maybe tuition reimbursement, small patient load or sufficient vacation time is the most important. Whatever you're important requirements, you should find out which employers will be able to supply them.

Don't be afraid to ask questions at the interview, you need to find out as much information about a place of employment as possible to make an informed decision. It's also good to know specific information about the area and the department as you can use it to guide your questions, your research also will impress the employer. If you interview with the actual unit, observe the interactions between the nurses, physicians, patients and others. This will enable you to get to know the atmosphere. Whether in a hospital or a different health care facility, ask questions of the nurses who work there, they are your best source of information.

Call or write potential employers and ask to talk with a personnel specialist or a specific specialty supervisor, radiologist, registered nurse, etc. who would be willing to talk to you in person about career opportunities. Briefly explain what you are interested in and ask if he/she would be willing to talk with you in person about career opportunities. If you are uncertain whether or not specific job skills are needed ask for the Personnel or Human Resources Department. This pre- interviewing is not always possible especially in a busy city hospital where staff members may not have the time to put aside to speak with a perspective employee.

For your informational interview bring a copy of your resume describing your desires and qualifications. Your resume must be in perfect form. If you need help, pay a professional to do them. This interview will help you investigate familiar and diverse employment opportunities. The outcome of these interviews will help you make an objective career decision and hopefully develop a company contact to help you land that perfect job.

When contacting people to request interviews add that you will only take 15 minutes of their time. Time is a critical resource that most of us use sparingly. If a supervisor's schedule is heavy you may suggest meeting them in the hospital cafeteria during lunch. Some healthcare workers need this rest period for themselves, but others use it as a social hour and may even introduce you to co-workers

During interviews ask specific questions to get the information you need. Here are some suggested questions:

> What experience/training is essential?
> How does my background compare?
> What advice would you give about this field?
> Does this company hire from this office or do they hire through a centralized personnel office?
> Is there advancement potential?
> What do you find the most and least enjoyable about this work?
> What type of additional training would I need?
> How did you personally prepare for this career?

You can also work with the classified and display ads in your local newspaper. Include national newspapers like the New York Times. Try special purpose periodicals, they provide classifieds for nurses also. Also, associations', newsletters, journals, Internet sites and other publications list employment opportunities and provide networking contacts. The Internet has changed the way job seekers access classified advertising. Many professional associations have employment ads on their web sites. Now more than ever there are excellent dedicated employment web sites with no fees for the prospective employee. Most notable among them are HotJobs.com, Monster.com and CareerBuilder.com. There really is a shortage of nurses and these web sites have many listings. Some healthcare facilities, businesses, and government organizations offer job hotlines. The charge for this service varies, but most are free. To find job hot lines, call the employment (human resources) departments of hospitals or local government agencies.

Job fairs are another source in getting the right position. They are usually conducted by trade organizations and provide direct contact with potential employers. Government organizations have placement services, they are sometimes referred to as resume matching services. Computers are often used to analyze resumes and match them to job vacancies. Healthcare associations can provide a wealth of valuable information when seeking a job.

Helpful Hints before entering Nursing are:
> Volunteer in a hospital or other healthcare facility to make sure nursing is the thing for you.
> Visit career fairs, to explore various career options in nursing.
> Shadow a nurse for a day.
> Join trade associations to obtain additional information on careers in nursing.
> Send your resume and cover letter to the Directors of Human Resources at local hospitals and healthcare facilities.

Where Are The Best Places To Work As A Nurse

There are advantages and disadvantages to wherever you decide to work as a nurse. About 60 percent of employed registered nurses, or 1.3 million, work in a hospital setting. About 17 percent or 360,000 nurses work in community or public health settings. In addition to the traditional hospital setting, nurses and nurse assistants work in nursing and personal care facilities, offices and clinics of physicians, offices and clinics of health practitioners (chiropractors, optometrists etc.), home care, kidney dialysis centers, drug treatment clinics, rehabilitation centers, blood banks, and schools, as well as general industry.

There are certain areas of nursing that may concern you more than others. You may be very concerned with the hazards of nursing such as the exposure to blood borne pathogens, like HIV, HBV, and air borne infectious diseases such as tuberculosis. Another major concern is exposure to chemicals, such as sterilizing agents and chemotherapy drugs. Particularly at risk are nurses who work in oncology departments. Nurses involved in direct patient care can suffer back strain from lifting patients and equipment. Home health nurses usually do not have the mechanical lifting equipment that are available in hospitals, so they are more at risk for back injury.

Some nurses have a shift work schedule that can cause a number of physical and psychological illnesses, such as gastrointestinal problems, exhaustion, depression, and anxiety. The frequent changing of sleeping and eating habits can disrupt family routine and social life. Others feel shift work can be a benefit when raising their children. Most licensed practical nurses in hospitals and nursing homes work a 40-hour week, some work nights, weekends and holidays. If you are the new nurse then you will have a good chance of getting an inconvenient shift. Most nursing position have eight hour shifts, however a department can elect to have twelve hour shifts. Twelve-hour shifts decrease your workweek to three days and can increase moral. Find out what shift schedule a department has to see if it fits your needs. Also in certain departments you can op to be on call if an emergency arises. This might be a good way of earning extra money.

Work place violence can be an issue depending where you work, but particularly for nurses who work in emergency rooms and psychiatric facilities. Nurses providing routine bedside care, may also help evaluate residents' needs, develop care plans, and supervise the care provided by nursing aides. In doctors' offices and clinics, they may also make appointments, keep records, and perform other clerical duties. Nurses who work in private homes may also prepare meals and teach family members simple nursing tasks.

You have to decide which concerns are the most significant to you. If your major concern is exposure to blood borne pathogens then working in a hospital with these types of patients is not the place for you. If concerns for exposure to chemicals were your major concern then working in an oncology department would not be good for you. You may have a weak back and lifting would be a major problem so you may not want to work in home care services. After you evaluated what your major concerns are you can choose what facility would be right for you.

Ask yourself these questions:

Do I want to work with patients that have HIV,HBV?

Do I want to work around sterilizing agents and chemotherapy?

Will I be able to lift patients?

Do I mind working the night shift?

Do I want to work in an environment where patients may get violent?

Do I want to work around electrical equipment?

Do I want to work with one doctor or many doctors?

Do I want to work with terminally ill patients?

Do I want to work with children?

Do I want to work with older patients?

After you answer these questions you will have a better idea of what type of healthcare facility you would want to work in.

Types Of Healthcare Facilities

There are many types of healthcare facilities. There are hospitals, nursing homes, doctors' offices, home and residential and hospice care services, schools and government agencies, clinics, and corporate research facilities.

Hospitals

Some form of institution for the care of the sick has existed longer than recorded history. The first centers for the ill were probably operated along with religious temples. The priest of these temples served as healers. A hospital is an institution that provides medical services for a community. They also try to prevent disease and maintain health throughout the community. In addition a hospital serves as a center for medical education and research.

The United State has about 7,000 hospitals and over 1,400,000 hospital beds. Each state has laws that a hospital must follow to receive a license to operate. The Joint Commission on Accreditation of Hospitals also approves most hospitals in the United States. Accredited hospitals must meet basic national standards established by the commission. They must also undergo periodic inspections.

Types of Hospitals

Every hospital is classified according to how long patients stay, kinds of services provided, and type of ownership. Most hospitals are short-term institutions in which the majority of patients stay less then 30 days. Patients spend an average of 6 to 10 days in a short-term hospital. In a long-term hospital most patients stay more then 30 days. People with mental illness for example would go to a long-term institution because of the time needed to treat such conditions.

A general hospital provides services for most people and for most types of illness. You will have scope of care, develop care for patient and developing nursing plans to abide by. A special hospital cares for certain persons or certain illnesses. For example, pediatric hospitals treat only children. A hospital may perform other services besides treating the sick. For example, research hospitals conduct various kinds of medical research and clinical trials. Teaching hospitals educate future physicians, nurses, and laboratory specialists and others planning a career in the medical field. A teaching hospital may form part of a university medical center, or it may be a general hospital associated with a medical school.

If you decide that a hospital is where you would like to work you will have to find the right hospital for you. Do you want to work in a public, private, or religious hospital? Each type of hospital has it's own philosophy of healthcare services. A religious hospital will have rules on life support and abortions issues. Public and Private hospitals will be more lenient with these types of situations. Where do your feelings fall on these issues and can you carry out the rules of the hospital on these issues even if you disagree with them?

Most hospitals are owned by their community, a board of trustees consisting of local residents manages such community hospitals in the public interest. A nonprofit voluntary hospital is owned by such organizations as charitable or religious groups. Community and nonprofit voluntary hospitals do not try to make a profit. They almost always spend more money for patient care than they receive in fees. Such hospitals must depend on donations. A private or proprietary hospital is operated like a business to make a profit for the owners. Several corporations own chains of short-term general hospitals. The federal, state, county or local government owns a government hospital. Hospitals that serve members of the armed forces their dependants, veterans, and Native American are examples of federally run hospitals. Some county and local hospitals operate like general community institutions and serve all the people in the area especially the poor.

Nursing Homes

Nursing homes are residential institutions that provide medical and non-medical care chiefly for people who are 65 years old or older. Nearly all nursing homes also accept younger patients. The best ones strive to provide a comfortable homelike environment for their residents.

The United States has about 19,000 nursing homes and about 1,300,000 men and women live in them. Most of the homes are privately owned while federal, state or local government operates others. Large corporations fund some private nursing homes, which try to make a profit for the owners. Others are sponsored by religious or civic organization, which do not try to make money. Each state has laws governing the operation of nursing homes and requires the institution to have a license. The homes are inspected periodically to make sure they follow these laws.

Types of Nursing Homes

There are three types of nursing homes: skilled nursing care homes, intermediate care facilities and supervised personal care homes. They differ according to the types of patients they care for and the kinds of services they offer.

Skilled nursing care homes provide more extensive services than the other types of nursing homes. They offer diagnostic, laboratory and medication services, therapy programs and dental care. Registered nurses supervise the care of patients according to the instructions of the institution's medical director. Physicians visit these homes frequently. Most patients require medical attention around the clock. Some have serious illnesses or disabilities. Many stay in these institutions after being hospitalized. Skilled nursing care homes are run by state licensed administrator.

Intermediate care facilities also called basic nursing care homes provide basic nursing services. Registered nurses examine the residents periodically to determine what treatment is needed. Most patients in intermediate care facilities suffer from a long-term illness. However they require only minor medical care. Doctors visit these nursing homes regularly. Registered nurses direct the nursing programs in intermediate care facilities, but administrators' runs these institutions.

Supervised personal care homes provide non-medical services. These services include preparing and serving the residents meals and helping them care for themselves. The members of the staff assist residents who have difficulty dressing themselves. The institution also plans social activities. Most residents of supervised personal care homes need only routine medical examinations and physicians visit these homes only when necessary. A supervisor of residential care directs the services provided.

Doctor's Offices

Doctors' offices can range from a very large complex of doctors and nurses to a single doctor rural office. They can be ambulatory care facilities, or day-op ambulatory care facilities. Nurses may assist in surgery and post op care of patient in these types of facilities. Depending on the community and the doctors, office conditions can be comfortable and well serviced. The duties of the nurse will depend on how the doctor she is working for envisions the nurse's role. Her duties can range from light to very heavy. Most of the duties involve routine patient care and check in preparation prior to the doctor's examination. The nurse may also assist in medical procedures that are done in the office.

Home and Residential and Hospice Care Services

In home healthcare, the nurse cares for their patients in the patient's home, a nursing home, or in the homes of their caregivers, so the work environment can be as varied as their patient's life styles. In addition, patients and family members can be under a lot of stress during this period and may be unpleasant and uncooperative at times. Some nurses are on call 24 hours a day and may be required to travel to homes in all neighborhoods of a city or in remote rural areas day and night. Safety may be an issue at times.

A Home Hospice nurse has to be comfortable in these situations. You have to ask yourself, "What would you do if your patient was in pain?" Suppose you couldn't contact the physician for a narcotic order? How would you manage? You still need doctors for medication, equipment orders etc. You have to be able and want to meet the needs of your patient at a critical time in their lives. You have to be able to coordinate everything that has to do with the patient's home care. If the family needs special equipment, such as a wheelchair or walker you will have to get it. You assess any symptoms related to the disease and take action. All hospice patients are expected to live less than six months and the majority die at home. Their needs are strictly nursing. They no longer can be cured. The patient's primary care is no longer given by a physician. As a Hospice nurse you can try to help the patients live the rest of their lives to the fullest. Hospice nurses are free to make their own decision about the patient. Some physicians' attitudes are, "If you can keep the family off my back, you can do absolutely anything within the bounds of safety.

Schools and Government Agencies

Community health nurses fall into this category. Most of these nurses work for government or private agencies. So do city, county, and state health departments employ nurses. Community health nurses may go into homes to care for patients who have just returned from hospitals. They often teach patients with chronic illnesses how to care for themselves. They also teach patients and their families about proper diet, personal cleanliness and other ways of preventing illness. Community health nurses may take part in many community projects some of them work in schools and camps.

Clinics

Clinics vary depending on the community. Some community clinics may be clean well-lighted buildings in upscale communities, while others may be in remote underdeveloped areas that have poor working conditions. Clinics are open to the community and the cross section of patients will be the image of the community. Working conditions in some clinics can be stressful when there are many patients and not enough staff to handle them. All types of patients are seen at clinics and there is a great diversity in patients' mental and physical situations.

Corporate Research Facilities

Corporate contacts offer an additional avenue of opportunity for the healthcare worker. Thousands of companies manufacture products or provide services to the medical profession. The major manufacturers have large research and development budgets and several operate healthcare facilities. Medical professionals, technicians, assistants and scientists staffs research facilities. Other positions include sales representatives who demonstrate complex systems and equipment. Corporations like these are always looking for salespeople with technical or medical backgrounds.

Interviews and Processing

Before you go into any interview, learn as much as you can about the institution where you are interviewing. Find out what their medical philosophy is. If they have a certain medical practice concentration in a specific area, become familiar with it before you go to the interview. This is where knowing someone in the institutions becomes helpful. Even if he doesn't have any power in the hiring process, he is a wealth of information about the policies and programs that are being used in that institution. Learn all you can about the institution and what they want their nurses to know and believe in so you can go to the interview with the same views.

Where you interview will usually determine how many people interview you. If you are interviewing in a one-doctor office you will only have to see him and decide if you can work with him. If you are seeking a position in a large hospital you will probably be interviewed by the charge nurses as well as some of your future peers to see if you would fit in with the unit. Getting a position in a large hospital especially a public one involves a lot of paper work and forms to fill out. The process may take awhile. In a small doctor's office or agency the process will be more streamlined. You will probably have to get a physical as well as a TB test for most positions.

Healthcare jobs are plentiful but they are still highly competitive. The more contacts you make the better your chances are to find the job you want. The importance of networking cannot be over emphasized.

Interviewers naturally have an opinion of whom the best candidate is after reviewing resumes and employment applications. Other employees who have had personal contact with any of the job applicants also influence them. I can't stress enough how important networking is.

The best technically or professionally qualified candidate may not get the position. Officials look at a wide range of issues, special skills, education, motivation, personality, and ability to get along with others. Through networking you give a positive image to the organization long before the interview.

Supervisors want motivated employees who can work independently, have the basic skills and training, and most important can get along with co-workers and patients. As long as you have the basics, don't be too concerned about others having more experience or training. If you show you are really interested in learning you may have the advantage over someone who gives the impression that they are a "Know it all". With the constant technological advances in healthcare, many supervisors know that employees who want to learn new skills will be a great asset.

Interviewers may ask you to tell the group about yourself. They purposely leave the question open to your interpretation. Many applicants limit their response to work experience and education. That is important but they already read your resume and know your professional background. Give them a brief overview of your education and experience and then lightly tell about your personal life and outside activities. This lets the interviewer see you as a person and not simply a candidate for the position. Make sure when you tell them about your outside interests it is positive and interesting.

For those who have already begun their career and are merely changing jobs, a popular question asked is: What did you like and dislike about your present or past employer? Remember no matter how you actually feel, be diplomatic. Employers are looking for employees who will support their organization not bring it down. If you negatively respond about your past or present employer it will only make you look bad. Your will be perceived as a difficult employee who doesn't get along in the workplace and then talks about how bad everyone is. For example a response to "What did you enjoy least about your past position?" would be: "I took work home but it took time away from my family, I resolved the conflict by devoting specific times during the a week to my family." This is a creative response indicating that you are motivated and can overcome the negative aspects. Don't badmouth previous managers or organizations. Any negative attitude will over shadow the interview and you will be perceived as a negative person. If you must talk about difficulties with a previous supervisor keep it to a minimum and be very tactful. Remember you are being interviewed by a supervisor who doesn't want you bad mouthing him at your next interview, he will also feel a little connection to the supervisor you are bad mouthing and may even know him.

Learn from the interview. If the person who interviewed you indicated that additional training would be helpful, look at what you need to do to get it. Try to learn from the questions they ask you during the interview. Did they ask you mostly about your experience, education or people related skills. You will always have to go for a physical and drug test if the position is offered to you.

Who gets the position is sometimes based on personality, positive attitude and motivation. There is a tendency to hire someone who is motivated but may have to be trained rather than hiring a problem worker who is well trained. Also, using these interview techniques to answering question will help you give a positive impression on an interview.

Conclusion

After reading this chapter, you now are more aware of why you want to be a nurse and the many reasons for choosing the nursing profession. It has enlightened you on what it is really like to be a nurse. You were given the opportunity to consider the many issues of nursing before you make your decision. A simple questionnaire helped you know your own goals. Now that you have examined your goals you have a better understanding of what you want and why. Ideas were discussed to enable you to become an effective nurse. Now you have a better understanding of why and what type of nurse you want to be.

Different types of health care facilities are outlined to give you a better understanding of nursing in every environment. Now you are aware of which institutions and salary levels would be best for you and how to obtain your ideal nursing job. This chapter also gave you helpful hints on what positions and institutions will be better for you. Helpful questions to ask yourself before applying for a position were given.

The interview and hiring process outlined in this chapter will help you know what to expect during any interview. If you follow the suggestions on how to find a nursing position, not only will you find the best position, it will be in the right institution also.

After reading this chapter you now know what nursing positions and what institution is right for you. You have a better understanding of the interview process and how to get the perfect nursing position for you. You will be confident knowing what position and institution is best for you.

Notes
1. Shelly Field, "Career Opportunities in Healthcare", (Checkmark Books 2002)
2. Ferguson's, "Careers in Focus Nursing", (Ferguson Publishing Company 2001)

Chapter 2

Salaries and Positions

The major occupational groups in nursing are Registered Nurses, Licensee Practical Nurses, Nursing Aides and Psychiatric Aides. There is a large range in salary depending on the position, education and training. Individuals often fail to negotiate a salary that reflects their intrinsic value and qualifications for the job. Knowing the normal salary range in your profession and in your location can be an important factor in easing into nursing.

A lot of people enter nursing for the rewards that the work promises, the prospect of healing people, the challenge of making patients well, and the personal satisfaction that good nursing yields. Nursing is inherently rewarding and self-sustaining with extrinsic rewards far less significant than in other lines of work.

However salaries and recognition are very important to nurses, and deprivation of both has demoralized nurses and discouraged people from entering the nursing profession. Nurses seek the salaries and recognition that make nursing financially possible and rewarding, thus signaling status and respect for the profession. Extrinsic rewards are more a means than an end in nursing, but they are certainly not irrelevant.

Nursing Salaries

Let's talk about nurses' salaries. If you are in a nursing position now, you know very well that you did not start out earning $60,000 a year, which a lot of people believe nurses start out with. You have to be working a good number of years before you get up to that level. Of course salaries differ depending on where you work and if you are a RN, LPN or an aide. RN's with a Bachelor of Science degrees start out with a higher salary than ones with Associates. There is differential pay depending on night or evening shift. You should try to enter an institution that meets your main financial needs. Even in the best situations RN's start at about $40,000, LPN at about $25,000 and aides at about $10.00 or less an hour.

Registered Nurses Salary

Median annual earning of registered nurses were $43,000 in 2002. The middle 50 percent earned between $38,000 and $49,000 a year. The lowest 10 percent earned less than $39,000 and the highest 10 percent earned more than $50,000 a year. Median annual earnings in the industries employing the largest numbers of registered nurses in 2002 were as follows: Personnel supply services $45,000, Hospitals $43,000, Home healthcare services $40,000, Offices and clinics of medical doctors $38,500, Nursing and personal care facilities $38,300. Nurse practitioners earned a low of $53,000 and a high of $80,000 the mean salary being $65,000.

Licensed Practical Nurses' Salary

Median annual earnings of licensed practical nurses were $27,000 in 2002. The middle 50 percent earned between $23,000 and $32,000 a year. The lowest 10 percent earned less than $20,000 and the highest 10 percent earned more than $37,000 a year.

Salary for Aides, Orderlies and Attendants

Median hourly earnings of nursing aides, orderlies and attendants were $8.00 in 2002. The middle 50 percent earned between $6.72 and $9.54 an hour. The lowest 10 percent earned less than $5.87 and the highest 10 percent earned more than $11.33 an hour. Median hourly earnings of psychiatric aides were $10.66 in 1998. The lowest 10 percent earned less than $6.87 and the highest 10 percent earned more than $15.28 an hour. Median hourly earnings of psychiatric aides in 2002 were $11.20 in State government and $9.80 in hospitals. Aides in hospitals generally receive at least 1 week paid vacation after 1 year of service. Paid holidays and sick leave, hospital and medical benefits, extra pay for late shift work, and pension plans are also available to many hospitals and some nursing home employees.

Registered Nursing

Registered nurses are the largest healthcare occupation, with over 2 million jobs, one of the 10 occupations projected to have the largest numbers of new jobs. The registered nurse's main purpose is to foster health, prevent disease, and help people deal with illness. They educate patients, families and communities. They provide direct patient care by observing, assessing, and recording symptoms, reactions and progress, assisting physicians during treatments and examinations, administering medications and assisting in convalescence and rehabilitation. RN's also manage nursing care plans, instruct patients and their families in proper care, and help individuals and groups take steps to improve or maintain good health. State laws decide which services RN 's can perform; it's usually the work place that determines their job duties.

Nurses who work in hospitals form the largest group. Most are staff nurses that provide bedside nursing care and carry out medical regimens. In this group of registered nurses there are charge nurses, nursing care coordinators (NCC), and Assistant Nursing care coordinators (ANCC). Also Care Managers are usually RN's who review the appropriateness of the patient's stay and speak with the doctor if they feel there is no medical necessity for keeping the patient as an inpatient. They give reviews to the managed care organizations (MCO's) and help arrange discharge, home care, and IV therapy at home. They may also supervise licensed practical nurses and aides. Hospital nurses usually are assigned to one area such as surgery, maternity, pediatrics, emergency room, intensive care, or treatment of cancer patients. Some may rotate through the departments.

Institutions that offer rotating job assignments will provide you with a broad range of experience before you consider specializing. Don't confuse this with "floating". Rotating programs are more formal, last longer and provided much needed training.

Office nurses care for outpatients in physicians' offices, clinics, and emergency medical centers. They prepare patients for and assist with examinations, administer injections and medications, dress wounds and incisions, assist with surgery, and maintain records. Some may include routine laboratory and office work as well.

Nursing home nurses manage nursing care for residents with a wide range of conditions. Although they usually spend most of their time on administrative and supervisory tasks, RN's also assess patients' medical conditions, develop treatment plans, supervise licensed practical nurses and nursing aides, and perform difficult procedures such as starting intravenous fluids. They also work in specialty care departments, such as long term rehabilitation units.

Home health nurses provide periodic services, prescribed by a physician, to patients at home. After assessing patients' home environments, they care for and instruct patients and their families. Home health nurses care for a broad range of patients, such as those recovering from illnesses and injuries, cancer, and childbirth. They must be able to work independently and may supervise home health aides.

Public health nurses work in government and private agencies and clinics, schools, retirement communities and other community settings. They focus on populations, working with individuals, groups, and families to improve the overall health of communities. They also work as partners with community leaders to plan and implement programs. Public health nurses instruct individuals, families, and other groups in health education, disease prevention, nutrition, and childcare. They arrange for immunization, blood pressure testing, and other health screening. These nurses also work with community leaders, teachers, parents and physicians in community health education.

Industrial nurses or occupational nurses provide nursing care at work sites to employees, customers, and others with minor injuries and illnesses. They provide emergency care, prepare accident reports, and arrange for further care if necessary. They also offer health counseling, assist with health examinations and inoculations, and assist to identify potential health or safety problems in the workplace in general.

Charge nurses or nurse supervisors direct nursing activities. They plan work schedules and assign duties to nurses and aides, provide or arrange for training, and visit patients to observe nurses and to insure that care is provided properly. They may also insure records are maintained and equipment and supplies are ordered.

Nurse Practitioners

The nurse practitioners are at an advanced level of nursing. They provide basic primary healthcare. They diagnose and treat common acute illnesses and injuries. Nurse practitioners can prescribe medications. Clinical nurse specialists, certified registered nurse anesthetists, and certified nurse midwives are all considered advanced level nurses. Advanced practice nurses meet higher educational and clinical practice requirements beyond the basic nursing education and licensing required of all RNs.

Careers Outside Traditional Nursing Settings

You can also take your career in a new direction. There are a variety of choices outside the traditional hospital setting. There are opportunities in Sales and Marketing, Nurse Outreach Educator, Nurse Recruiter, Military Nurse, Medical Writer/Editor, Flight Nurse, entrepreneur Consultant, Traveling Nurse, Nurse Informatics, Holistic Nurse, Forensic Nurse and Legal Nurse Consultant.

In sales and marketing positions a nurse promotes pharmaceutical/medical products and services. You must maintain a relationship with clients, customer service and participate in trade shows. A background in sales/marketing is useful. Some companies rely mainly on inside sales people. You would be going to the office every day and your main customer contacts will be by telephone. Other companies favor outside sales people. There you will have an opportunity to work from home with a flexible schedule. Travel is often required. If you're inclined to get into sales try both inside and outside sales to find which you prefer. You will usually find you are better at one versus the other.

Some companies prefer college graduates. Potential employers include pharmaceutical companies, medical supply companies and telephone marketing companies.

The nurse outreach educator works in hospitals, clinics, social services offices and educational institutions. As an outreach educator you conduct seminars, and counseling sessions as an advocate for health issues. You should be able to communicate well in groups, and have good writing skills. A bachelor's degree/RN and experience working in social services or education is usually required.

As a nurse recruiter you contact and place nurses in jobs at healthcare facilities. It involves selling placement services to nurses. You should have an excellent phone voice, be positive and enthusiastic and be able to develop a rapport with candidates. Communication and interpersonal skills are essential. A bachelor's degree is usually preferred. Employment opportunities are with travel healthcare companies, staffing agencies, hospitals; convalescent care centers and other healthcare facilities.

A military nurse has all the duties of a traditional nurse during both war and peacetime settings. During wartime she may be given a wider range of responsibility. She may be classified as active duty, reserve or as a civilian employee. An RN/BSN enters active military duty as an officer. A military nurse can be called for global wartime duty, sent overseas or into service in combat hospital units. There can be a long time commitment for active duty and reserves. Some military nurses return home apparently fine but the repercussions of war and trauma frequently catches up to them in their personal lives later on. Usually a military nurse has critical care, and/or trauma experience. A RN with a bachelor in nursing is required for active duty, but not mandatory in the reserves or civilian employment.

A medical writer/editor works in all aspects of writing and editing of technical material. This material is used in research, education, training, sales and marketing. You will have opportunities for freelance work combining writing skills with medical knowledge. A bachelor's degree or higher is usually required. Hospitals, medical marketing/communications companies, pharmaceutical companies, medical trade journals and other publishing companies employ medical writers/editors.

A flight nurse deals with emergency and non-emergency air/surface transport of sick and injured patients. She should have critical care experience as well as strong communication skills. Education requirements are an RN with Advanced Cardiac Life Support Certification and Pediatric Advance Life Support Certification. Flight nurses are employed by trauma centers and other acute care facilities, public and private transport companies and the military.

An entrepreneur is a person who starts his own business and who assumes all the risks and responsibilities associated with it. A consultant is an individual who provides expert services on an hourly basis. Either may work in any area of the healthcare/medical industry. Required skills include a well-rounded education and a creative risk taking personality.

The traveling nurse works on temporary assignments. These assignments are from eight to twenty-six weeks, the average being thirteen weeks. As a traveling nurse you can work on a cruise ship or have a resort position. They often work in exciting cities in top facilities and earn top dollar. Expenses are paid by the travel companies, and include housing, health insurance and travel reimbursement. You should have a good clinical background and adapt and make friends easily and get along with all types of people. Educational requirements vary, although most traveling nurse are RN's.

A nurse informatics position involves all aspects of computerization related to nursing and healthcare practices. This includes data analysis, system management, software design, training, systems installation, sales, marketing and medical library work. The main requirement is knowledge of computers and software. Degree programs are offered but not required. Positions are available in healthcare facilities, computer hardware/software companies, educational institutions, regulatory agencies, pharmaceutical/research facilities and healthcare consulting firms.

Holistic nurses are involved with treating the whole person rather than just the disease. It is the mind, body and spirit approach. Backgrounds for this position include massage therapy, acupuncture, educator, and trainer. A holistic nurse is interested in the wellness, healing and preventive medicine from a spiritual and more natural view point .Certification and or licensing may be required. It varies from state to state. Positions are found in healthcare facilities, holistic health centers, health clubs, resorts and spas, in private practice, pain treatment centers and physicians' offices.

The forensic nurse combines clinical nursing practice with law enforcement. She is involved with investigation and treatment of victims. As a forensic nurse you will combine nursing knowledge with investigative skills. Certification for forensic nursing is usually required. Forensic nurses work at healthcare facilities, correctional institutions, county prosecutor and coroner's offices, medical examiners, insurance companies and psychiatric facilities.

Legal nurse consultants are nurses who usually work for lawyers or insurance companies that review patient cases that are filed for medical law suits. They help determine the course of action and severity of the suit. Legal courses are usually required for this position and the pay is somewhat lower then other nursing positions.

Nurse Practitioners and Physician Assistants

A physician assistant works under the direct supervision of a specific physician and usually takes medical histories, conducts physical examinations, orders lab tests, changes dressing, performs minor procedures, and counsels and educate patients on health matters. Like the nurse practitioner the focus of the physician assistant is wellness. In rural areas nurse practitioners and physician assistants have played a major role. There is a push for nurse practitioners to assume a greater responsibility such as writing prescriptions and admitting patients to hospitals. Both nurse practitioners and physician assistants require additional college studies. Local medical centers or colleges/universities can provide this.

The role of these two positions has caused conflict between the American Medical Association and the American Nurses Association. The idea of nurses writing prescriptions and the prospect of nurses receiving direct reimbursement from insurance companies have some doctors upset. Doctors may perceive this extension of duties as an infringement on their closely guarded world. Some do not want to give up this control.

Rehabilitation Nursing

The world of rehabilitation is fast becoming the career of the future. With the baby boomers getting older and the increase in sports activity in general, this area of nursing is on the rise. Rehabilitation nursing will be a thriving specialty in the very near future. Master's degrees in rehabilitative nursing are being offered in universities throughout the United States.

Nurses Aides

Nurses aides are the backbone of long term care facilities and hospitals. They perform a difficult and sometimes thankless job. A nurses aide is expected to be a cheerful jack of all trades for very little compensation. It's is a hard job with long hours. They perform direct personal care for the patient such as baths, linen changes, toileting assistance, hygiene and feeding.

Part Time Work

If part time work is a consideration you may want to look into Home health nursing, Clinic nursing or Physician's office nursing. You may find a position in home health nursing through a home health agency. Clinical nursing at urgent care centers , walk in clinics and ambulatory care centers may offer flexible scheduling options especially if you are able to work evenings. In Physician's office nursing you may also be able to find part time hours.

Conclusion

There are many different positions in nursing. This chapter helped you find the right one. It exposed you to the many facets of nursing and the salaries involved. The most well known is the registered nurse, practical nurse and nurses aid. Salaries depend on the nursing position, education, experience, location, and facility you work in. It is important for you to do your homework and find which nursing position fills your needs.

Nursing is a personally rewarding career but salaries can be an important factor also. Nurses seek salaries and recognition that make nursing financially possible and rewarding. It is important for you to do your homework and find out what the average salary is for your type of nursing position in order to successfully ease into nursing. You can easily find this out through your college, employment agency, newspaper ads, or friends and family in the health field. Usually once each year, medical journals publish salary comparisons for many types of positions. These can be found at your local library.

Registered nurses usually start out with a salary of about $43,000. Licensed Practical Nurses make about $26,000 and aides about $10.00 an hour. Nurse practitioners average about $65,000. Registered nurses are the largest population of nurses. They provide direct patient care with the most possibility for advancement. As a registered nurse you can work in a hospital, office, nursing home, patient home care, public health services, or industry.

There are also many careers outside the traditional nursing profession. This chapter has given you insight into some of these new and exciting opportunities in nursing. There is the traveling nurse for those interested in seeing new and exciting places. There is the nurse informatics, who are involved in all aspects of computerization related to nursing and healthcare. This chapter has outlined some usual as well as unusually vocations in nursing while giving you some idea of salary. Now you should have a better idea of what position would be right for you.

Chapter 3

Schooling, Policies and Procedures

Most nursing schools admit only candidates for registered nurses who rank in the upper half or upper third of their high school graduating class. Entrance qualifications for practical nursing are less stringent. High school graduates are preferred, but many practical nursing schools accept applicants with two years of high school or less. Usually nursing schools admit students from the age of 17 on.

The cost of a nursing education program varies with the school. Hospital schools require entrance fees and charge tuition. In colleges of nursing, students pay tuition. Nurse loan repayment programs help recruit and retain nurse. By taking a position with a facility and pledging to work a certain length of time you can get a loan repaid by the facility. These nurse loan repayment programs are about partnerships between colleges, health systems and in some cases partnerships between middle and high schools.

Professional and technical education

There are two types of entry-level nurses: Licensed practical nurses (LPNs) and registered nurses (RNs). LPNs attend a 12 to 18 months vocational training program then take the NCLEX-PN, the national licensing exam for LPNs. RNs complete either an associate's or bachelor's degree of science in nursing, then take the NCLEX-RN, the national licensing exam for RN's. There are also three year hospital based diploma programs (non degree granting) for RN's. These programs qualify applicants to take the NCLEX-RN as well, but are few and far between. Financial aid is available for both LPN and RN programs.

Nationwide data show that 61 percent of new registered nurses come from associate-degree programs, 36 percent from bachelor's degree programs and 3 percent from hospital diploma programs. The demands of modern day nursing require a more educated nurse work force because hospitalized patients tend to be sicker and treatments more complex than in days past.

Associate degree programs consist of a two-year course of study in nursing care and related subjects. Many junior and community colleges offer such programs. Students also gain practical experience by working in a local hospital and other health agencies that cooperate in the programs.

Diploma programs are offered at hospital schools. They require two or three years of study, after which the student receives a diploma. Students take nursing courses in classrooms and laboratories and they work with patients in the hospital and at health agencies.

Baccalaureate programs offered by colleges and universities lead to a Bachelor of Science degree. The course work requires four to five years. It includes training and experience with patients in hospitals and health agencies as well as courses in nursing, science and the humanities. These nursing education programs provide both classroom training and practical experience. They prepare the student for obtaining a license to practice as a Registered Nurse. In most university programs nurses are being reared alongside the physicians in medical schools and so they have the opportunity to interact with physicians and develop skills in important critical circumstances.

Student nurses study such subjects as anatomy, chemistry, nutrition, pharmacology, physiology, psychology, and sociology as well as the fundamental of nursing care. They learn to care for the sick by working in the nursing laboratory. Students also learn by practicing on one another.

Please make certain that any degree you obtain is in nursing, especially when going back to school for advancement. Many nurses make the mistake of obtaining non-nursing degrees and then become frustrated when their careers do not advance.

Two Year, Four Year and Diploma RN Programs

The debate over two years, four-year and diploma RN programs has been raging for many years. And has caused much controversy. The question is, in the real world will you receive less professional respect if you have a two year degree.

Here are some facts: Two year RNs take the same licensing exam as four year RNs. Two year RNs take most of the same classes and have similar clinical experiences during nursing school as four year RNs, the difference generally being a broader liberal arts foundation and added coursework in the area of research and management for the four year program. Both enjoy the same scope of practice unless you live in South Dakota, where a BSN is the minimum for RN licensure). The difference in pay, if there is any (and often times there is not) is typically less than $1,50 an hour. The difference at this time seems to relate to career mobility and advancement. If you plan to go into management, the BSN (four-year degree) is the better way to go. If your long-term goals are to advance practice or specialty certification, a BSN will be necessary as will a master's degree. There are many programs to help you achieve a BSN or MSN later on, if that is your goal.Generally there is little differentiation between two and four year RNs once you go out into the working force. Respect will come based on your performance and knowledge and skills you bring to the job, not your degree. With the current nursing shortage, this should not be an issue in terms of employment.

How to Choose a School

When finding a nursing program the first thing to do is check the basics. It should be accredited by either, the National League of Nursing's Accrediting Commission or the Commission on Collegiate nursing Education. Also verify that the nursing program is approved by your state's Board of Nursing or Department of Education. Making sure your nursing program is accredited and approved ensures that you will qualify for the licensing exam and that your licenses will transfer to other states. Some factors to look for when comparing programs are:

What is the NCLEX examination pass rate?

What percentage of students each year go to graduate school?

What type of support services are offered through each program?

Are there any major differences in the program?

These factors will help you decide which program actively encourages and supports students, thus enabling academic and clinical success.

Best Education For You

The next step is to find which program will provide the best fit for you. Some programs will just fit better with your personal circumstances, goals and finances. It is a very personal decision when it comes to which degree would be best for you. It really depends on your situation in life and your career goals. It is always desirable to get the highest degree but this may not be possible at first. If you are changing your career to nursing and you all ready have a BA you may feel differently then some one just starting out that has no degrees. You may choose a two-year program because it's fast and you can find facilities where the degree doesn't influence the pay as much.

Also you may have to take into consideration whether you can afford to go to school for four years. Two-year program will be less expensive and after you start working at a hospital you have a good chance of getting them to pay for the rest of your education. Of course getting your desired degree at the start can be the best way to go. But if this is not possible there are many ways of gradually achieving your goals depending on your situation. Find the path to nursing that fits your current needs. Nursing school is tough, no matter which program you choose but you will be able to successfully find the right program for you.

Some helpful suggestion to find the right program for you are: *What is the overall cost for your education at the school in question? What financial aid options are available at the school? What is the average class size? What are the typical program hours? Is the program highly structured or flexible?*

Finally to get a truly unbiased opinion, talk to the student nurses themselves. What do they like about the program? What do they dislike? Do they feel they getting a quality education? Would they recommend their school?

Selecting a nursing program is a highly personal choice based on many factors. You need to evaluate each program and choose the program that will work best for you.

Registered Nurse

After graduation from an approved school of nursing, students must pass a written examination. The nurse then receives a license to practice in that state. He or she is now a registered nurse (RN). Depending on the state you may have to take courses to renew your license every few years. Nurses may advance their careers by additional study and experience. A master's degree is often the step to specialization, teaching or administration. To advance further a nurse may earn a doctoral degree in preparation for teaching and conducting research.

Practical Nursing Courses

Practical Nursing courses usually last one year. Like professional and technical nursing educations, practical nursing courses combine classroom study with hands on experience. There are two types of practical nursing programs, public and private. Some public schools teach practical nursing as part of their vocational training or adult education programs. Private schools are operated by hospitals, health agencies and by some junior colleges and universities. Credits for courses taken at vocational nursing schools cannot be directly transferred to professional or technical nursing schools. Some nursing school programs allow vocational nurses to obtain a degree without repeating basic courses.

In all states, a practical nurse must obtain a license to practice in that state. He or she then becomes a Licensed Practical Nurse (LPN, sometimes called a Licensed Vocational Nurse (LVN).

Advancement, Training and Other Qualifications

Students must graduate from a nursing program and pass a national licensing examination to obtain a nursing license in all states. Nurses may be licensed in more than one state, either by examination or endorsement of a license issued by another state. Licenses must be periodically renewed. Some states require continuing education for license renewal.

In 2000 there were over 2,200 entry-level R.N programs. About one fourth of all programs offer degrees at the bachelor's level. About 4 percent of hospitals offer diploma level degrees. Generally, licensed graduates of any of the three program types qualify for entry-level positions as staff nurses.

There have been attempts to raise the educational requirements for an R.N. license and maybe create new job descriptions. These changes, should they come about will be made by each state. Changes in licensing requirements would not affect current licensed RN's, who would be "grandfathered in". Individuals considering nursing should take these changes into consideration when deciding to enroll in a Bachelor's program, since they will have more advancement opportunities. Many career paths are open only to nurses with bachelors' or advanced degrees. A bachelor's degree is usually necessary for administrative positions and is a prerequisite for admission to graduate nursing programs.

Many diploma-trained nurses enter bachelor's programs to prepare for a broader scope of nursing practice. They can often find a hospital position and then take advantage of tuition reimbursement programs to work toward a Bachelor's.

Experience and good performance can lead to promotion and more responsibilities. You can advance, into management and become assistant charge nurse, or charge nurse. From there, you can advance to assistant director, director, and vice president. Management level nursing positions require a graduate degree in nursing or health services administration. They also require leadership, negotiation skills, and good judgement. Nurses can choose a path to become a clinical nurse specialist, nurse practitioner, certified nurse-midwife, or certified registered nurse anesthetist. These positions require one or two years of graduate education, leading in most instances to a master's degree, or certificate.

Some nurses move into the business side of healthcare. Their nursing expertise and experience on a healthcare team enables them to manage ambulatory, acute home health and chronic care services. Healthcare corporations employ some nurses in health planning and development, marketing, and quality assurance. Other nurses work as college and university faculty or do research.

Internships/Preceptorship

Most health care facilities provide the novice nurse with an internship program followed by a preceptorship. Novice nurses may receive a 7 week nurse internship program, while critical care novice nurses may receive a 10 week nurse internship program. After the internship, novice nurses then progress to a unit specific orientation with a preceptor. A preceptorship is similar to a one-on-one with a clinical instructor. Preceptors are always at your side, making sure you know what you're doing and why you're doing it. Preceptors take new hires and provide in-depth orientation to unit operations and any education not covered in a nursing textbook.

It takes a special type of nurse to take on the responsibility of showing new nurse the complexities of a specialty area. A good preceptor must have good communication skills, a lot of patience, strong clinical experience and knowledge. They are also excellent resources for any questions you have. You and your preceptor should be paired together for several weeks, to ensure learning what you will need for success. After your preceptorship is over you are the nurse and you will be responsible for the care of your patients, even if it's something your preceptor didn't cover with you.

During this time the key to success is asking questions. Try to avoid being the know it all novice nurse or the novice nurse who lacks confidence. No one expects you to graduate nursing school and be the super nurse who knows everything. Nor do they expect you to graduate nursing school with little knowledge or confidence. You are expected to have adequate knowledge and confidence in your ability. Also be receptive to new ideas and information, because you will learn more in these few short weeks then you ever could imagine.

Quality

Quality is what a patient wants and what the nurse wants to give. Florence Nightingale first did quality assurance back in the 1850's. She established quality standards that were fairly basic. She told the generals, "Our soldiers are in more danger from being in the hospital than if they were fighting on the battlefield. You'd better shape up." They did. Her recommendations for hospital management were based on her statistics on the outcomes of hospitalized patients.

That is what quality assurance is. You figure out what you think you want, go out and measure what you have and then take action. Unfortunately quality assurance in the health field right now is ninety percent political and ten percent methodological. The federal government Diagnostic Related Groups and Professional Review Organizations control consumption of health resources and label it quality assurance.

Quality is now being looked at by many regulatory agencies who are making sure that quality data and patient outcomes are being regulated. There are now many internet report cards that can find out data regarding quality in hospitals.

Some people in the medical profession want to drop the assurance section. They don't want to be responsible for assuring quality especially with the high cost. So the Federal Professional Review Standards substituted the word, "assessment" instead of, "assurance". This means they only check to see if standards are met. Professional Review Organizations are supposed to be accountable for quality. What they do is pick two or three commonly seen medical diagnoses and look at the kind of medical care that goes into that type of patient. No explicit nursing is considered. Nurses are caught in the middle of this. Nurses know what quality care is and yet the system's isn't setup to carry out that quality.

From Florence Nightingale's time right up until now, thousands of studies have been conducted, and standards developed based on those studies. There is the Nurse Standard of Care, which every nurse learns in school and practices in every department that they work in. Yet the standards may not help us understand the problems of quality achievement. The nurse will assess the patient and arrive at a nursing diagnosis. It is just the beginning of the standards that acknowledge nursing diagnosis. The more knowledge nurses assess and diagnose, the larger the number of ways to take care of patients. As a nurse you will have to obtain realistic views on quality. They will have to include the institution's standards and definitions according to their cost efficient ways. This is not what a new nurse wants to hear but it is what you have to acknowledge.

Policies

Even after you get the required schooling for whatever kind of nurse you decide to be you will have to learn the policies of the nursing profession in order to succeed. Many nurses feel it is the system that is the problem and may make them want to leave nursing. The lack of appreciation by the nurses you work with, superiors and the power plays of the physicians and how they try to put the nurses against each other can be an issue. Even after you have established good working relationships with physicians, they seem to do things to protect themselves or get the better end of the deal. It could be an endless power struggle. Become aware of this and protect yourself, don't be naive and think the physicians are going to always be fair with you.

Physicians sometimes feel they don't have much control over the system either. Things may get delayed. The doctor may get frustrated by the slow down and blame the nurses for foul-ups in the system. They may threaten to bring in physician's assistants so they can have the same kind of control they have in their private offices practices. This can be frustrating to a nurse.

This next story about the opening of a bone marrow unit portrays polices and procedures you may encounter as a nurse. A bone marrow unit was started before it was ready. Policies and procedures should have been in place before it opened, but supervisors at a high level were involved in the decision to start the unit early. The head physician was very aggressive, and he wanted the unit opened. A few nurses protested acknowledging the fact that because of the lack of organization there would be staffing and patient problems. The old guilt trip was stated "All those patients are out there ready for transplants and they may die if we can't do them." The real reason was money. The hospital would double its income with the new unit and they didn't have to hire more people.

At first it went fairly well with a small work group. Then, other people came in who started to question the policies because they'd been hastily put together. The head physician wasn't around much, so there was little support when problems arose in the very new program. Staff nurses started to feel frustrated and unappreciated. Physicians started telling the charge nurse how to staff her unit. Nursing administration started going along with it, and the physicians got their way. They weren't looking at what this was doing to staff morale or the quality of care in the unit. Try to protect yourself from this situation. Beware of new department openings; they may be too much for a new nurse to handle. Try to find your first job in an established unit or department where you know there is support.

Procedures

Sometimes with federal regulations as they are certain constraints are placed on the healthcare facilities that causes real ethical problems for the nurses working there. For instance, it is important to have a certain, "Payer mix" if the health facility is going to stay making a profit. Private patients subsidize the cost of patients on Medicare, so you need to reduce the Medicare admissions and increase the private payers. This is hard to do because you have to turn away some needy patients on Medicare. It is illegal to turn away any needy patients on Medicare. You will encounter this turmoil no matter where you work; it is just a fact of life. Try to find a facility that has this to the degree you can cope with. All patients are supposed to be treated equally but this is not always the case.

If an institution starts to have fiscal problems, administrators handle them by reducing staff. You will still have the same number of patients but they will expect the nurses that are left to do more work for the same pay and with fewer resources. This is a stressful situation. The best way to avoid this is to find out what the budget and money situation is at the institution before you accept the position. If budget cuts develop while you are there and it becomes too stressful, then it might be time to look for another position.

Hospitals are Businesses

Hospitals, like all other businesses must make money in order to stay alive. Metropolitan areas once had many independent healthcare facilities. Because of spiraling healthcare costs and the burden of more stringent government regulations, many of these facilities have had to close their doors or have been merged into larger corporate conglomerates. Even today, these large corporate hospitals are finding it difficult to stay afloat.

As hospitals struggle under various financial and government obligations, nurses are sometimes caught in the middle. They can be worked to death and the burnout rate is soaring. It is ironic that amidst all the layoffs and restructuring there is still a nursing shortage.

Nurses who have been able to keep their jobs have had to endure ever-increasing workloads in order for the hospitals to maintain their economic balance.

Competition among certain hospitals is serious. To remain competitive hospitals obtain the latest in equipment and technology. They then try to reduce cost and increase profits. Hospital stays have been decreasing ever since Medicare came out with DRGs (Diagnosis Related Groups) The focus is now on out patient care and reduced staff or downsizing.

In-House Pool and Floating

To compensate for downsizing, hospitals have developed in-house pool and floating positions. In house pool provides an incentive for nurses to work additional hours or shifts. Nurses are offered more money per hour to work more. It is hoped that this will encourage employees to work extra time therefore eliminating the need to hire additional nurses and pay the benefits or resort to the use of expensive nursing agencies. Floating is when a nurse from one unit is put temporarily in another unit where she may not have the knowledge or expertise needed to give the best care. A nurse from a medical floor may be sent to a Coronary Care unit.

When asked to "float" to a new unfamiliar area you should assess the situation. Try to think of it as an opportunity to learn new skills, but if you are uncomfortable talk to your supervisor and try to make other arrangements. Negotiate a safe floating situation if you can. Maybe submit a "protest of assignment" form and make a private notation of the occurrence in a diary or journal. Ask your co-workers how they best handle uncomfortable floating situations. Also when one unit is over staffed and another is under staffed a nurse is "pulled" to the understaffed unit. Try to avoid going to a unit you feel you can't handle. Unless you have an agreement you will probably be obliged to, "Float". This is not what you want to hear about but it is what you will find when you work at a hospital. Luckily, in most hospitals floating is not used to any great extent. Try to find out how extensive this practice is and decided if you can be comfortable with this situation.

Nurse Practice Act

States have Nurse Practice Acts, which allow review of legal functions of nursing. Nurses mounted a campaign to see that educationally qualified nurses could be allowed to practice nursing outside direct control of the physicians. Nurses have some very strong opponents in the medical community. Physicians feel they need to be in control. The Nurse Practice Act tries to convey what nursing diagnosis is. Physicians seem to have no concept of this. They feel the word diagnosis is theirs. It's also an economic thing. Physicians were having problems with people dictating to them how they will practice. When they learned that nurses wanted to insert nursing diagnosis in the Nurse Practice Act, they figured this is one thing they could curtail. Nurses are required to know a lot of what doctors know but doctors don't understand the nurse's education. It's unfortunate, but that's been the history between doctors and nurses Doctors and nurses should work together but unfortunately this is not always the case. So nurses have their work cut out for them and you will have your work cut out for you as a new nurse. But you can accomplish a happy medium between you and the doctors. Just do your homework and find the institution that has the most similar views as yours. Then within that institution find the best department for your needs.

American Nurses Association and National League of Nursing

The best way to be politically aware is to join and become active in a nursing organization. On the national level, there is the American Nurses Association and the National League of Nursing. In addition each state has its own organizations, which serve it's immediate membership. Most nursing specialties also have their own organizations. They work at national and state levels to lobby for the bills that will effect nursing. They also publish journals and newsletters that will provide you with valuable information. These associations provide a sense of professionalism while uniting nurses under a common cause.

The American Nurses Association is interested in national issues. It works toward unifying the legions of nurses, working or retired throughout the United States. It works through the state nursing associations striving for strong educational programs and lobbying of state and congressional legislators to pass bills that will help nurses. The ANA's main source of information is the American Journal of Nursing.

The National League of Nursing is a nationwide educational organization. It offers libraries, videos and books for continuing education. It strives to keep nurses informed of current practices and looks for changes that might better the nursing profession.

In 1893 the American Society of Superintendents of Training Schools for Nurses was started. This was the first organization for nursing in the United States. The society was formed for the establishment and maintenance of a universal standard of training for nursing. In 1912 it was named the National League for Nursing Education (NLNE). In 1917 it released the first Standard Curriculum for Schools of Nursing. In 1952 the NLNE, the National Organization for Public Health and the Association of

Collegiate Schools of Nursing established the National League for Nursing (NLN). Membership is available to nurses interested in nursing education as well as public members. The National League for Nursing Accrediting Commission (NLNAC) was established in 1997 and is responsible for all accrediting activities and is accountable to the NLN directly through the NLN's Board of Governors.

The American Nurses Association (ANA) became involved in collective bargaining in 1946. Key issues were nurses working over 40 hours a week and nurses receiving $.78 an hour while other women in the work force were making $.95 an hour. Nurses did not have any benefits. Nursing was regarded as a dedicated calling, not an economic pursuit. Collective bargaining is a tool for addressing workplace concerns. The ANA has been involved in issues such as equal pay for equal work as early as the 1940's.

In 1999 the ANA formed the United American Nurses (UAN), a formal union of nurses. The Union for Nurses is comprised of Constituent Member Associations (CMA) of the state nurses associations involved in collective bargaining. The UAN represents more registered nurses than any other union. Nurses know what the nursing issues are. The UAN helps nurses advocate for nurses so that nurses can advocate for patients.

ANA has been recognized for a 100 years as the voice of nursing. The UAN has instant creditability and resources and access to the right decision makers. Working with the UAN, nurses are able to protect themselves from work related hazards, learn their rights and enforce the laws that protect them. Nursing practice and quality of care issues are top priorities for the UAN.

If you really want to become involved you can usually do so within the hospital where you work by joining a committee. Not all hospitals have unions and even if the hospital where you work has a union your joining it is usually optional You have to decide how important it is for you to work for a union affiliated hospital. You might also seek out seats on the hospital board. Also you can become involved politically at the local level to make your voice heard. All these things should be done after you have been in your position for awhile. Don't start to become politically involved too soon. Give yourself time to find out how your supervisors feel about politically involved workers.

History of Nursing

Florence Nightingale gave us the first taste of the nursing profession. She set her sights to make nursing an honorable and respectable profession. Women were regarded as naturals for a calling that required sensitivity and warmth. In the early part of the 19th century women preformed private nursing duties in the home such as childbirth, terminal illness, care, etc.

Before the 1870's there were no trained nurses. Some upper class women who were appalled by the existing hospital conditions recognized the need to train nurses and established nursing schools. Interestingly, at the time, doctors were resistant to educating women in nursing. Other more affluent men such as bankers, lawyers, and businessmen assisted in raising money to build decent hospitals and start nursing schools.

The first three nursing schools were established, in the United States, by 1873. By 1900 there were 432 nursing schools and 1,192 by 1910. These schools were the training grounds for middle class women who wished to work outside the home. Nursing courses were associated with hospitals. The diploma programs took three years to complete and in most cases included boarding at the school. These programs were strictly for women who wanted to be nurses, no college courses were offered.

By WW II nurses found conditions and pay in the military superior to civilian nursing positions. In 1946, civilian staff nurses were earning less money than typists and seamstresses. This produced a nursing shortage which led to the development of one-year education program for practical nurses (LPN) or licensed vocational nurses (LVN).

The first university-nursing program was established in 1909 at the University of Minnesota. By around 1960 the Bachelor of Science degree in nursing was the norm. Then two year registered nurse programs became available at junior colleges thus the Associate in Arts degree. Degrees in one, two, three and four years were now available to women who wished to become nurses. Nursing schools had the choice of accepting the brightest applicants.

Men started to filter into nursing after the Vietnam War. The war had produced corpsmen who had medical training. Nursing offered these men an opportunity to begin a new career when they came home from the war.

Conclusion

In order to cope with the issues in the nursing profession you will have to learn the policies and procedures of the institution where you work. Nurses have to sell their preventive services to the institutions that are concerned about money. You have to demonstrate savings through prevention. Only then, the hospitals, the Federal government, and industry are interested. So the nurse has to make alliances, plain and simply based on the value of their worth. As a new nurse you will have to learn how to accept this.

You may have a conflict within yourself when you become a nurse on the issues of, "What should I be doing as opposed to what the institutional values are". Sometimes you will find yourself doing what the institution wants you to do as opposed to what you believe you ought to be doing. There may be a difference between your values and the polices and practices of the institution where you work. No one wants to tell you this but this conflict does exist and you will have to learn to deal with it when you become a nurse. If you accept that there will be a conflict no matter where you work you can then find the place that has the least amount of conflicting issues and work there. Find out about polices and procedures of the institution before you accept the position. Talk to friends and family who are associated with the institution and can give you insight into the issues.

In this chapter you have learned the different educational requirements for whatever nursing field you choose to go into. Nurse degrees are offered by two-year community colleges, three-year hospital diploma programs and four-year Bachelor of Science programs. Findings have suggested that nurses with four-year bachelor's degrees instead of just two or three years of education may lead to substantial improvements in quality care. You were provided with information on the requirements for certain positions and advancement.

Quality of patient's care was discussed and how quality assurance and assessment is being monitored. You now realize how nurses can get caught up in quality assurance issues and how to protect yourself. You have been enlightened on the physicians' role toward nurses and the Nurse Practice Act. You have learned how to not be naive and protect yourself.

As a nurse you can be shaping your future rather then waiting for the institution to do it. If you combined the ideas of "what ought to be" with "what is" you can figure out where you want to work and what you want to do as a nurse. The hints outlined in this chapter will help you understand the policies and practices of any institution that you work in. You are now more aware of what you might encounter and how to handle each situation. The essence of nursing is really the concern for patients. Nurses often do everything for their patients and that will never be measured in dollars and cents.

Chapter 4

Administrators, Physicians, Charge Nurses and Managers

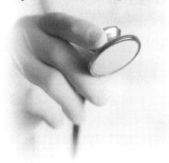

Here are some hints that will help you as a beginning nurse make sense of the social world you might encounter at the institution where you will be working. The health facility is a hierarchical social system that you have to accept. Almost at the top of this hierarchical system is the charge nurse. At the top come the administrators and board of trustees or the owner. There are higher positions, such as the state health department, federal government health regulations departments' etc., but they are distant from the immediate life of a nurse. The structure that usually affects the nurses day-to day life looks something like this:

Administrators/Board of Trustees or Owner
Department Heads/Supervisors
Nursing Director
Nurse Managers/Nurse Care Coordinators
Assistant Nurse Manager/Assistant Nursing Care Coodinators
Charge Nurse
Registered /Staff Nurses
Practical Nurses
Nurses Aids
Patients
Families

Most hospitals have an administrator who is responsible for the operation of the entire institution. The board of trustees or the owner appoints this official. In some cases, a private management firm provides the overall administration of the hospital.

Various departments handle a hospital's business affairs. Each department has a Department Head. There are many departments in a hospital such as the administration office, business office, purchasing and facility departments, etc. The admitting office schedules patients for admission at the request of their physician and assigns them to rooms. The business office lists each patient's charges, prepares a bill at the time of discharge and records payments received. The purchasing department manages a hospital's stockroom and buys supplies and equipment. Facility departments are responsible for the buildings and grounds as well as management and disposal of biological and hazardous waste materials.

Most hospitals have units, each of which cares for certain groups of patients. The number of units varies according to the size and type of hospital. In large teaching hospitals physicians are usually the heads of the departments. Not all hospitals have physicians as heads of departments. Also a nurse supervisor will be in charge of the nurses in these units. There are usually three supervisors, morning, evening, night that reflect the three shifts of the hospital. Most general hospitals have several basic units. For instance, the maternity unit helps protect mothers and newborn babies from infection by keeping them apart from other patients. Except in extremely small hospitals, children stay in a pediatric unit designed especially for their needs. Some hospitals also have a teen-age unit. Men and women who do not require surgery stay in the adult unit.

The surgical unit cares for patients awaiting surgery or recovering from an operation. Most hospitals also have a recovery unit in which patients who has received a general anesthetic can be watched closely after surgery. Some hospitals have a psychiatric unit for mentally ill patients. A few have separate units for burn victims, heart patients, premature babies, and others who require special care. Most hospital units are intermediate care units, in which the professional staff gives patients constant care and observation.

Intensive care units serve critically ill or injured patients. The intensive care unit because of the severity of the patients can be the most stressful unit for a nurse. It can have the most burnout and turn over of nurses.

Some hospitals have minimal care units for patients who are well enough so that they or their families can provide much of the nursing care needed. A few institutions have parent care units for children. There a parent stays with the child and provides all nursing care except technical treatments. A hospital also has an emergency unit that provides care for accident victims and persons who have suddenly become ill or injured

Physician-Nurse Relationship

Most physicians have an office practice and send their patients to the hospital when necessary. Physicians are usually associated with a single hospital.They then supervise the hospital treatment. In all hospitals there are some physicians who work directly for the institution and do not have a private practice. These doctors may include such specialists as radiologists, who direct a hospital's X-ray services. In some hospitals, many or all members of the medical staff work directly for the hospital. This arrangement occurs chiefly in government and university hospitals and in hospitals operated by labor unions or other groups for the benefit of their members.

The nurses' relationship with the physicians can vary considerably depending on the personalities of the physicians, nurses, and the institution that they are working in. The department or unit that you are in can also influence these relationships. Some departments have a history of physicians treating nurses a certain way. It could run from treating you with respect to being treated like you were a servant. Nurses usually work directly with the attending physicians. You have to do your homework and find out the practice of the unit before you accept a position. In most cases there is a healthy equal co-worker type relationship between doctor and nurse. A small percentage of unequal situations do exist and you must become aware of this. Like in any business, there are good employers to work for and there are poor ones.

In the past, the relationship between doctors and nurses was similar to that of a father and daughter or husband and wife. The wise physician kept a protective wing around the naïve women nurse. These roles were shaped by gender and training. These roles do still exist to a small extent but have been altered considerably. Today you can no longer assume a doctor is a man and a nurse is a woman. At least, 38% of students graduating from medical school are women.

In medicine, woman physicians have to fight for their rights. They know the difficulties of being a woman in a world overrun by men. You will find most women physicians respectful and know how helpful nurses can be.

If you decide to confront a physician you have to be very careful how and where you do it, otherwise, the physician may retaliate on you or the patient. You have to also be careful about not getting in between a patient and a physician. An example of this is, a pregnant woman who refuses an enema, and her physician gets mad and delays starting the Pitocin to induce labor. He was angry because the patient had defied his orders, so he decided she'd have to wait. The nurse knew this physician; if she confronted the physician with his defiant behavior at that crucial time the patient would have received the brunt of his anger. So she decided to stay quiet. You will have to learn how to read physicians personalities in order to protect yourself and your patient.

In institutions where there is shared governance, both physicians and nurses get together periodically and clarify their roles and develop procedures. Some institutions don't have this, then the physician has a lot of power and the hospital is giving the doctors even more say, just to keep them there. In this type of setting the nurse has to learn to read the physician's personality traits in order to know the best way of handling each situation.

Nurses juggle a lot of personalities and preferences. A unit will work differently depending on which nurse is on duty. Nurses who are openly assertive are labeled aggressive. Once the physicians label you aggressive, no one wants to work with you. You lost your credibility. You can continue to be assertive and insist on doing nursing things, but the physicians will challenge every decision you make. So be careful how you go about getting your nursing done. Do it in a way that doesn't irritate the physician. Try to first handle problems yourself before going to the charge nurse or nurse manager for help. Sometimes talking to the doctor or asking fellow workers how they handled similar situations can help you solve the problem.

Some of the problems with physicians are due to nursing managers who fail to support their staff nurses. When a physician confronts the nurse manager, shouting, "Can you believe what your nursing staff is doing!" the manager had better be strong, and secure enough in her own position to confront him back or she is incapable of defending her nursing staff's actions. By caving in to every physician's criticisms or even whims, a manager is limiting the respect her nurses will be getting in the future from these physicians.

Some believe physicians try to control nurses' practices because they feel threatened. Maybe if nurses demand their practice rights, the patients might realize that most of what they need is nursing. Another real fear of the physician is a malpractice suit. If roles aren't clear-cut and something adverse occurs due to a nurse's action, the physician may be held accountable. Social policy may need to be redefined to clearly give the nurse responsibility and authority for her actions.

In most cases you will find that doctors and nurses respect each other. Doctors are the bosses but usually they work with nurses in an equal co- worker relationship. The few cases where doctors mistreat nurses are something you should be aware of and try to avoid. They are the exception not the rule but you still must become aware that they do exist so you can avoid these unfair situation. Don't be naïve, protect yourself.

Interns

Physicians also include intern and residents physicians in training. They have graduated from medical school and work in a hospital for required on the job experience. Learning goes on between the residents, physicians, and the nurses. The residents don't resent this: they depend on the nurses to help understand the particular protocol of an attending physician. It takes time to learn the individual physician's likes and dislikes. The resident will count on the nurse to clue him in. You might find yourself directing the resident on the medical treatment for a very sick person. It is the nurse's job to call the patient's physician if you think the resident physician is using poor judgement. For example you may think the patient is retaining too much water. If the resident doesn't take action you will have to call the physician directly. Attending physicians expect the nurses to alert them in situations like this.

Here is a story about a nurse and a physician's relationship. Sue's first job was as a nurse practitioner, she worked with patients in a hypertension clinic. She was part of an experimental program sponsored by the Department of Preventive Medicine of the local medical college. Her job responsibilities were to set up and administer the clinic. She carried out the medical plan independently, unless there was a problem. Everyone seemed to be happy with the arrangement, including the physicians.

The clinic hired nurses, rather then physicians, primarily because of the cost. It was cheaper to have nurses do the job. Sue was getting a nurse's salary for doing many of a doctor's tasks. For about a year and a half everything went well. Then a physician, an internist from another department, came in. He was upset with what Sue was doing. He said, "A nurse shouldn't be doing what Sue was doing". It was just an excuse to get her out. In reality, he wanted his medical students to work in the clinic, so he bumped Sue from the clinic. Medical students are free help, so he didn't need a nurse practitioner any longer.

Since the hospital had a union, they couldn't fire her so administration transferred her to the emergency room. The medical director was disheartened to lose her but when push came to shove, he went along with his colleagues. Sue pleaded with the nursing supervisor to petition the union but the nursing superior didn't want to make waves. She told her, "Leave well enough alone - you are getting paid - you still have a job."

Most of the time you will not be in this situation. But there are a few times when you will find this. Try to protect yourself. Try not to put yourself in an unstable position where you are vulnerable to physician's whims. Look at the position realistically before you accept it.

Supervisors Nurse Service Director;Manager, and Nursing Staff

Heading up the entire nursing program in hospitals are the Supervisors, Nursing Service Director and Nurse Managers/Nursing Care Coordinators, who administer the nursing, program to maintain the hospital's standards of patient care. The Nursing Services Director advises the medical staff, department heads and the hospital administrators in matters relating to nursing services and helps prepare the department budget. They may be in charge of hiring and firing their staff, as well as evaluating their performance. They are usually responsible for maintaining patient and department records. They may be responsible for developing and maintaining budgets. Nursing Managers are often in charge of establishing, implementing and enforcing departmental policies and evaluation the nursing staff. Some nurse managers provide nursing care to patients along with managing the department or unit.

The nursing staff forms the largest group on the patient care team. Charge nurses are in charge of the nursing staff in that unit or department. Registered nurses carry out much of the patients' care under the direction of physicians. Registered nurses also direct other members of the nursing staff, including practical nurses, nurses' aids and nurse attendants. These men and women do many routine, but necessary tasks that free the registered nurse for work requiring their special skills.

Nurse managers/Charge Nurses-Nurse Relationships

Many people interact within a health institution: Nurses have many relationships within an institution. Some of these relationships would be; Registered nurse manager nurse, registered nurse assistant manager nurse, registered nurse-charge nurse, registered nurse-registered nurse, registered nurse-nurse practitioner, nurse-physician, nurse-resident, nurse-patient, nurse-family of patients', etc. Any experienced nurse can tell you none of these relationships has a greater effect on the quality of life in a health institution than the relationship between a nurse and the charge nurse. The best characteristic of a good unit is a healthy nurse-charge nurse relationship. If the nurse-charge nurse relationship can be characterized as helpful, supportive, trusting and revealing of knowledge, then it will be a wonderful atmosphere in which to work. The relationship between nurse and charge nurse seems to have an extraordinary effect. It models how all relationships will be. Your charge nurse will convey her opinion about you to the nurse managers who probably do your evaluations.

You want to get into an institution where the charge nurse-nurse relationships are supportive, close, helpful, trusting and stable. The new nurse has to learn to understand the views of the charge nurse. For example if the charge nurse is very child oriented and allows parents to stay with their very sick children you will have to have that view and follow through with it. You have to start to learn the views, needs, and wants of the charge nurse even at your own expense, so that you can achieve harmony in the workplace.

New nurses have to be concerned with the same issues as the charge nurse, and they have to want to solve them in the same way as the charge nurse. If you make the charge nurse's job easier then he/she will like you and want you in their unit. On the other hand, as a RN you have an obligation at some important times to confront managers if need be and not just go with the flow. Just do it very diplomatically and only when absolutely necessary. See chapter 9 on how to successfully complain for when you feel you must confront a supervisor.

Nurse Managers and Assistant Nurse Managers

There are many different types of nurse managers. Each person will handle the responsibility in a different way. Maybe the manager took on too much and doesn't know how to handle the problems in the department. Some managers may forget where they came from. They may forget what it was like to be a nurse. In the beginning she may want to right all the wrongs but then in face to face combat with administration she loses. Or she may feel threaten by a more knowledgeable nurse she has to manage.

Some nurse managers will use their power as a weapon rather than a tool. Their attitude may be, " I'm the manager and I can do whatever I want and you'll do as I tell you." Their thinking may be if I was treated that way, now that I have some power I'm going to get my revenge. For other nurse managers, control is everything. They may already be closet control freaks and in this position of authority control runs rampant.

Some nurse managers are threatened by a department where everyone gets along so they play one employee against another. Some nurse managers take a negative approach and tell employees only about the negative aspects of their work performance. Then there are nurse managers who think the world of their nurses and let them know they're appreciated.

We must not forget the male nurse manager. They make up a small percentage of the nurse manager population but they are an important part of the system, Male nurse managers may fit into the supervisor, physician relationship easily. They may be more likely to resolve differences between male physicians at a local bar or sports event. Working under a male nurse manager can have its advantages. Do your homework and find out if a male nurse manager is right for you.

The charge nurse-nurse relationship is one in which the supervisor has more control, power, and the upper hand. Many Charge nurses view themselves as the policymakers of the unit and view the nurses as executives whose task it is to make that policy operational. A real affiliation problem can arise when the charge nurse holds this view and a nurse doesn't.

Most nurse managers will be a combination of these types of personality to varying degrees. Try to find out what personalities a charge nurse is more prone toward before working in that department, this way you can find the one you may be most compatible with.

Nurses are dependent on their supervisor for keeping their positions, for promotions, for references, and for various favors such as certain working schedules, and evaluation, etc. Many nurses express concern because supervisors seem to make important judgments about them, their patients and their families on a limited amount of information. Increased contact with the charge nurse can help you identify the expectations of your supervisor. But if the charge nurse is leaving you alone and seems to be happy with what you are doing then leave well enough alone.

Task Versus Relationship

Charge nurses, nursing service directors or managers, physicians, department heads or administrators, who are in leadership roles, are either task- oriented people or relationship- oriented people. The task oriented administrator derives major need satisfaction from the successful completion of the task. The relationship-oriented administrator derives basic need satisfaction from successful interpersonal interactions. The task-oriented person might expect reports to be completed, patients to demonstrate progress, supplies to be ordered, etc. A relationship-oriented leader will place a higher value on the morale and camaraderie that exists among the staff, how well they work as a team, or on having warm relationships with their patients. Most managers exhibit both sets of leadership qualities but tend to place a higher value on one versus the other.

Some desires a charge nurse might exhibit to her nurses will include some combination of the following:

Wants to keep staff members at a professional distance.
Does not want to become too involved in the personal lives of staff members.
Wants staff members to be task-oriented and not spend too much time socializing and discussing unrelated subjects.
Does not want to get too close to the staff because their evaluation should be as objective as possible.
Wants to be able to rely on his/her staff for help on any project.

The nurse's expectation of the charge nurse could easily include any combination of the following:

Wants to get to know the charge nurse as more than just a robot professional.
Would like to be able to talk to the charge nurse and have the same goals.
Wants to know what the charge nurse expects of her.
Wants to be able to rely on the charge nurse for support.
Would like to be on a friendly basis with the charge nurse.

The expectations that a charge nurse and nurse have effect their communication and understanding of common goals. Problems may arise because of differences in expectations. It is important for a new nurse to become enlightened on the expectations of the charge nurse.

It is true that supervisors deserve the employees they have. Once a supervisor observes unacceptable behavior or performance, it's his or her responsibility to counsel the employee immediately to correct the deficiency. The primary goal of the supervisor is to improve the employees' performance or behavior. It's unfortunate that many supervisors go to great lengths to avoid constructive confrontation and often ignore behavior and or performance problems until they get out of control. This is a disservice to the employee and to the organization.

Charge Nurse's Favorites

Even a fair charge nurse may have her favorites, but as long as she is not downright mean to anyone and she supports her nurses, you can work under her. That's important. If you have a charge nurse who takes her nurse's side, then you have a good chance of succeeding.

Most supervisors have their favorites and usually they are the nurses who have been there the longest. Sometimes they worked with these nurses before they were supervisors. When the supervisor first came to the ward, she relied on the nurse's who had been there the longest for information. These nurses may have told her about everyone and everything. They are the nurses who usually do the extras for the supervisors when they don't have to. They are the ones the supervisors know they can rely on for favors. They might be the nurses who tell the supervisors the gossip about all the other nurses. The nurses who talk about everyone to the supervisor are usually the supervisor's favorites. They don't complain to the supervisors. They give information their own way. This might sound upsetting to you, but it is what you need to know to survive in your positions as a nurse.

Sometimes in a hospital there will be a lot of nurses like this. They can be like ladies-in-waiting around the supervisors. Only they may be managers-in-waiting. For instance, a charge nurse, a very nice person, worked with a few of the experienced nurses and they now tell her every little piece of gossip. If these managers-in-waiting do not like you, you can be sure that in a little while the charge nurse will not like you either. When you get unto a unit, it shouldn't take you long to discover which nurses are the supervisor's favorites. When you first get into the ward, they will be the nurses you want to complain about to your supervisor. They are the nurses who are telling you what you should and shouldn't do, and they are the ones that might not be doing their own job properly. But, of course, you can't complain about anyone. Complaining usually back-fires for a new nurse. Be nice to them, accept their advice, and try to stay on their good side.

Fair Charge Nurses

Above all you must work under a fair charge nurse. Nothing is more important than that. If a charge nurse wants you in her unit, you are there. If the charge nurse doesn't want you, you are gone. It's as simple as that; there is no other way of putting it. If you get a charge nurse who is fair to everyone, and if you do your job the way she wants you to, then you will have a position there. But, if you get a charge nurse who is not fair and she decides you are not what she wants on her floor for whatever reason, and it could be for the most bizarre reason – you will not be there. It might be because you don't have the same perspective about solving problems as she does. Find out, and try to acquire the same problem solving skills as the charge nurse.

How to Find a Fair Charge Nurse

More often than not newly starting nurses do not have the luxury of choosing their charge nurse or Nursing Care Coordinator or Assistant Nursing Care Coordinator for they just begin work in the department they were hired for. There are a few things you can do to find a fair one. First do your homework before you go for the position. Find out as much as you can from family and friends about the position. This is where networking is helpful, you will not be going into a position cold, you will have some resources for information about the position and the managers.. Sometimes asking other nurses who have worked under her will give you a better answer

However, nurses who are working under a charge nurse at the present time may not be able to tell the truth about her for fear of losing their positions. If they are being harassed by the charge nurse, and have decided to leave, then they will be able to talk. The most reliable sources are the people who left. They will now tell you if the charge nurse has harassed them and others into leaving. If two different sources tell you the same thing about a charge nurse, take it as truth. You couldn't get better information, and at all costs, don't work under that charge nurse. Unfortunately, it is very difficult to find people to talk to who have already left the institution.

The charge nurse is the almighty on any floor. Protect yourself. Work under a fair charge nurse, because no one will or can help you if you find yourself working for an unfair one. Don't be naïve and think that everyone is fair and there is no such thing as an unfair charge nurse.

Most charge nurses are fair and you will be able to please them, the odds are in your favor when you get a position. Just be a little cautious at first, cooperate with the charge nurse, and you shouldn't have any problems. This advice is not what most people are comfortable conveying to the new nurse, but it is what every new nurse should know and everyone is afraid to tell them.

Here is a story about one of those managers-in-waiting, a registered nurse named Mrs. Silver, who had been in the unit forever and knew everything about the department. The charge nurse relied on her to organize charts, order supplies and do other supervisory tasks. Mrs. Silver would have something to say to the charge nurse about everyone and everything. She was very bossy to the new people, telling them what they should and shouldn't do, as though she were a supervisor. For example, she would tell a new nurse little things such as how to fill in certain entries on charts and how to handle a patient. You had to obey. God forbid if you said something negative to her or disobeyed her.

She would report back to the charge nurse and soon the charge nurse would be looking at you and wondering. You had to learn to get along with her, but if you couldn't, then you had to keep out of her way or at least stay on her good side when you had to work with her. The next year she was promoted to a charge nurse position in a different unit. She was now an official supervisor! If in the future you found yourself working for her at least you had a good history. This juggling takes a lot of humility. But if you want to be a successful nurse, this is what you will find yourself doing.

You will always find bossy experienced registered nurses in a department. They will be more than ready to tell you what to do and will report back to the supervisors on your level of obedience. So beware, be careful, be humble, and be obedient. Treat them like supervisors. They may really be trying to help you in their own way, and if you don't obey them they can cause trouble for you. They don't have the title of supervisor but they act as if they do. Be careful of them and try your best not to alienate them. Don't fight with them; try to avoid them if they really get on your nerves. They have experience and connections on their side, and your are not going to win if you buck them, so don't. This is what no one wants to tell you when you start your career in nursing. You usually have to find this out for yourself the hard way. But, of course, not all nurses are like this. There are many experienced nurses who are genuinely friendly and helpful.

Experienced Nurses

You will receive an orientation when you start a new position. Some experienced nurses feel it is their responsibility to assist incoming nurses who may be novices. They work with them, befriend them, answer questions, and anticipate areas where they might need help. Most of the time these are very nice nurses who really want to help you. On occasion you may find a nurse who has other reasons for wanting to help you. You have to make sure your relationship stays one of informal assistance rather than formal supervision.

Many nurses comment that they learn from training others. Assisting others in the craft of nursing can be an attractive and rewarding experience for some, unless the surrounding circumstances make it inconvenient or burdensome.

Nurses Who Give Advice

Advice can be very helpful when it is just that; advice. When it becomes a command then it can become troublesome. There are some nurses who put their two cents worth of advice into everything and it can be very annoying. You may wonder if they do it because they want to be helpful or because they are just naturally bossy. Either way, you have to deal with them in a cordial manner. They probably want to be helpful, and this is the only way they know how.

There is a type of registered nurse who falls into this category. She will stop you in the hall to say that your charts are fine but you wrote the procedures different then the way she does and you shouldn't leave them that way. First ask yourself, "Who is she to tell people what should be written on patients' charts? Is her title chart nurse? When she tells you things like this you are not sure if she is trying to be helpful or bossy. Then ask yourself, What should I do? Should I change the chart? If she is not a supervisor and no supervisor requested the change, why make the change? The best thing to do with a nurse like that is to say, "Thank you very much" and do whatever you want and not worry about it unless a supervisor says something to you.

If you do what such a person suggests, whether you agree with it or not, you run the risk of reinforcing her bossiness and she might tell you what to do more often. Of course, if she is very chummy with a supervisor, and tells the supervisor about it, you may have the supervisor on your back. However, she may genuinely be trying to help you by telling you before a supervisor does. You have to decide what the real motive is and act accordingly.

Who Do You Obey?

Choose carefully which nurses to obey. Try to find out which ones go to a supervisor if their suggestions are not taken. With this bossy one, the new nurse chose to take the chance and did not make the changes to the patient's chart.

In another instance a new nurse first came to the unit and an experienced registered nurse told her all sorts of things to do. The new nurse started to get annoyed. The experienced registered nurse came to the new nurse in the main station and asked why she was having certain things done for a patient. Who was she that the new nurse had to explain why she wanted something done for a patient. So the new nurse nicely told her not to worry about what she had to do. If the supervisors had a problem with what she was doing they could talk to her about it. The experience registered nurse didn't like this, but she backed off and didn't try to give the new nurse advice for awhile.

Be careful in the beginning who you listen to; you may be making some nurse your boss without realizing it or wanting to. You don't need or want any extra bosses. Try not to make enemies either. You never know who will become your supervisor in the future, because occasionally, it's one of these bossy experienced registered nurses.

Beware of nurses who break hospital rules and expect you to do the same. If a nurse wants to break hospital rules let them do it alone. Protect yourself; you don't know if anyone else will. Don't let another nurse bring you along when they are breaking the rules, especially when you know it's one of the charge nurse's pet peeves. You can't afford to be culpable when rules are being broken. That could easily be grounds for dismissal. Experienced nurses can get away with more then others. As a new nurse you must follow every one of the charge nurse's rules to the fullest. You don't want to get a charge nurse on your back just because you annoyed her by breaching her rules.

Only when absolutely necessary ask other nurses for favors. If you ask others to take your call or to work your Saturday shift you are now obligated to them. You will have to reciprocate. This can be a way of forming a bond but if done to often or if one becomes unsatisfied it can become a source of conflict. As a new nurse you should try to keep this practice to a minimum.

Please don't get the wrong impression; most nurses are genuinely friendly and nice. Don't isolate yourself from the staff. New nurses are far more likely to achieve success when they find colleagues to help them through the uncertainties and hazards of patient care, etc. Just pick carefully which nurses you have help you and how.

Male Nurses

While only 6.2% of practicing nurses are male, more men are finding nursing an appealing profession. Although salaries are not high, nursing offers stability and mobility and extra shifts can help financial needs. Following the Vietnam War, men who were trained as medics often turned to nursing. Since that time nursing programs have seen an increase in male enrollment. Male nurses add another dimension to medicine. They fit easily into the good old boy network. As in the business world it is not unusual for male nurses, especially senior staffs nurses or nurse managers and male physicians to resolve their differences and reach understandings on the golf course or local bar. At times this camaraderie extends to sales representatives from medical supply companies. You may find working under a male senior staff nurse more to your liking.

Diverse Staff

Most people achieve genuine intimacy with only a few people in their lifetime. You are not likely to bond with those significantly different from yourself, but it is crucial that you understand the role they play in your world. The staff of a hospital is not usually a band of similar people but offers a rather wide range of different and diverse personalities that make up a healthy hospital staff. It is a society where people would not naturally experience intimacy with each other, but none the less learn to share a common territory and common values for the sake of the whole institution.

Although the extent and intensity of staff interaction vary widely for nurses, the threat of isolation is ever present and the benefits of congenial interaction are by far more beneficial. Most nurses value productive institutional interaction and would like more attention to this in their contacts with peers. The more diversified the staff the more difficult interaction becomes. A large city public hospital will have the most diversity among the staff. This diversity usually diminishes as the size of the hospital decreases. The smaller public hospitals will have a more uniform staff while private and religious hospitals will have the most homogeneous staff.

Every department, floor, unit or ward has its own personality. Some hospital's personnel will be more compatible with your personality than others. There are hospitals that have an all for one, one for all team spirit among the staff. Then there are hospitals that are not so congenial and may have cliques that divide the staff.

Fellow nurses also offer recognition for good nursing and peer praise is highly valued. The understanding acceptance of colleagues and their continuing support mitigate the isolation that you might otherwise experience on the job.

Humor is another tool that will help bring together a diversified staff. If you can see the humor in a situation this will help. Every staff can find common situations to laugh together about. Bring humor into you interactions with staff members.

Evaluations

Many people and situations effect your evaluation. Your co-workers can be friendly with the charge nurse and tell her how they feel about you and this will effect your evaluation. The charge nurse obviously has a say in your evaluation and the nurse manager or assistant nurse manager will probably be the one to write your evaluations.

First you have to develop a good rapport with your fellow workers especially the nurses that have been there a long time, The next major step is to develop a good working relationship with the charge nurse. Then your relationships with the nurse managers or assistant nurse managers are already half won over. If the nurse managers are hearing good things about you from the staff and charge nurse you will more then likely get a good evaluation from them. Just make sure you know what the nurse managers want you doing and do it.

Building A Support System

How do you perceive support? Do you give support as well as accept it? Supportive charge nurses, nurses, doctors, aids and administrative staff are important to your easing into a nursing position. When you do get a nursing position, the following are some questions that might help you learn how you deal with getting support. Answer each question with the name of a person you would most likely go to. If you would solve it yourself, write no one.

If you had a bad day and wanted to talk, to whom would you go to?
If you needed help giving medication, to whom would you go to?
If you needed to know more about a patient, to whom would you go to?
If you really disliked a patient, to whom would you go to?
If you thought a group of nurses were treating you unfairly, to whom would you go to?
If you needed help with a chart, to whom would you go to?
If you were angry with another nurse, to whom would you go to for advice?
If you thought the charge nurse was harassing you, to whom would you go to?
If you thought one of your patients were misdiagnosed to whom would you go?
If you had trouble with a patient, to whom would you go to?
If you had a patient's family member who was particularly troublesome, to whom would you go to?
If you were able to help a patient in a special way, to whom would go to?
If one of your patients did unusually well, to whom would you go to?
If your supervisor gave you a compliment on your work with a particular patient to whom would you go to?
If you found a new and better way of doing a procedure, to whom would you go to?

Check your answers. Do you have a lot of "No one" answers? If you have more then five you might want to think about adding more people to your support system. Remember everyone needs other people, because you can't do everything by yourself. Also, do you use one person's name frequently? If so, you may be depending on that person too much. Are you reciprocating? Remember you are part of other people's support systems. They may be the beginning of friendships and they may be part of the group you will fit in with at the hospital. So set up some time to nurture the relationships with these people with whom you feel comfortable.

Work Friends

When making friends at work, you must be careful. There are friends and then there are friends from work. You may find that if a person has to choose between a friendship formed at work or maintaining a job, nine times out of ten he or she will pick the job. People are there for the job, especially if they have mortgages or rent, loans, children in college, etc. Everyone wants to be friendly, but when push comes to shove, a job is wanted or needed more then a friendship. If all of a sudden the charge nurse didn't like you, and there is a threat you'll be out of a job soon, you would be shocked at how fast most of your work friends will treat you differently, as if you had the plague. They will be afraid to be around you for fear of becoming associated with you and also losing their job. It is not easy for a charge nurse to get rid of a nurse due to personality but it can happen. I know this is a little disheartening but it is a reality of nursing that no one wants to tell you. Nursing has been described as the only profession that eats its young. So don't be naive, protect yourself.

Inexperienced Nurse

Here is an example of an inexperienced nurse's plight in an unfriendly hospital unit. Try to avoid this state of affairs. One new nurse; we will call her Polly, worked in a hospital in the suburbs. Everything was fine for the first year. The nursing service director and charge nurse loved her. The nurses she worked with loved her and she loved them and her job. Then the Charge nurse left and all hell broke loose. There were budget cuts. A lot of people were shifted to different departments. She found there was no one left whom she knew or knew her. The new charge nurse inherited Polly. She made it clear from the moment Poly stepped onto her floor that she did not want her there. The charge nurse harassed her from the moment she started till the day she had enough evidence to fire her. Everything was done legally.

First, she tried to intimidate Polly into quitting. She wrote horrible evaluation after horrible evaluation stating she was sending them to the main office. Polly found out later that the charge nurse never sent them to the main office. She was telling Polly that to pressure her into resigning. Obviously the charge nurse didn't want Polly there. Maybe she had someone else in mind for the position. Polly never found out the real reason. The charge nurse did the same thing to the next nurse, and she got away with it again, but this time the nurse was experienced so she was only transferred to a different department instead of being fired.

When word got out that the charge nurse was dissatisfied with Polly, no one wanted to be around her. This charge nurse had a history of harassing workers, but the people who worked there did not take the side of the harassed workers. They all looked out for themselves.

The union representative was as supportive as she could be, but legally the union could only help if Polly were experienced. If you are experienced you have already proved yourself as a nurse so the union can fight back with your past history. If you are inexperienced, the union cannot help you if a charge nurse is harassing you.

This situation is not the norm, but it does happen. Most likely you will never find this extreme situation in your hospital, but it does exist, and it may be there to some extent in any hospital. You have to learn to protect yourself. Work under a fair charge nurse and cooperate with him or her. Understand that you need friends at work but realize in what context and to what extent. It is understandable that people will place their job at a higher priority than friendship. So, find your comfortable level of interaction. This is something no one is going to tell you at work but it does exist.

Nurses-Nurses' Aids

As a nurse you will have to get along well with the nurse's aides and L.P.N.s.. Don't ever ask them to do something you wouldn't do yourself. Their help is vital to the running of the unit. If you get on their bad side you can find yourself making beds and fetching food trays. The nurses' aids' power and effectiveness usually reside in their relationships with people in the community. They can be relatives of patients in the hospital or have a strong bond with the community in some other way. As a new nurse you can learn a lot about the patients and the community from them. They can get the word out to the community very quickly about the new nurse. Since the way you treat them becomes the way you treat the whole community, treat them well.

Colleague Interaction

Most people are innately considerate and respectful to their fellow workers. Colleagues are important in meeting your social needs for adult contact and support; they are the primary source of advice and emotional support. Many nurses like to share their techniques and ideas. You will find some nurses who are more than willing to share their good ideas with you. Most nurses both initiate and welcome exchange of ideas and emotional support.

When you are starting out, you will find a need at some point to search for emotional support and new methods for your patients' handling. Improving your own nursing skills is always important. Since there is an interdependent character to nursing, cooperation with colleagues is vital for emotional support and methods.

Colleagues also participate in setting and upholding standards for good nursing. Open and continuous exchange among staff is most likely to promote a consistent set of standards that will make nursing easier for you.

There may be times however when you are faced with an uncooperative group of colleagues. When this negative situation occurs look at the possibly reasons.

Is your peer support level set too high.
Are you sensitive to the nurse's time
Are they extending to you the same respect and courtesy they wish to receive.
Are they burnt out

Whatever the cause may be you must continue to act professionally, take care of yourself and try to get along as best you can. You might want to take a direct approach and deal with the situation head on. Some passive aggressive bulling behavior tends to evaporate when it is confronted rationally, calmly and assertively. It may even open a dialogue.

Don't let a bad experience discourage you, it is the exception not the norm. Most nurses are friendly and helpful to newcomers in the unit.

The Nurses' Role In The Social Order

Being a nurse is being smack in the middle of the social system of the hospital. The patients and their families are underneath, and the administrators and all the bureaucrats at the main office, as well as the hospital board, are above. The nurse is subject to demands from below and directives from above. A nurse who becomes too close to the patients or aides is looked upon as lower in the social order, while one too close to the administration is considered a climber. However discontented some nurses may be with the social system as a whole, they obey certain rules in order to protect their status and maintain some solidarity as a group, no matter how much internal tension there might be among them. Some of the rules are:

Don't criticize or outwardly disagree with another nurse in front of a patient or their family members.

Don't criticize another nurse at a staff meeting.

Don't talk about other nurses to a patient or even to anyone else when a patient may be in earshot.

Talk to another nurse privately about a problem.

Try not to say anything derogatory about another nurse.

Choose your clique of nurses at the hospital, and eat lunch with them.

Don't try to change the procedures a charge nurse or department has put in place.

Don't do any part of another nurse's job unless you are asked to by her or a supervisor.

Don't complain to a supervisor about another nurse.

Reciprocate any favors that are given you.

These rules serve to present a unity among the staff before the patients, their families, and administrators. New nurses who do not observe these rules to some degree will be looked upon as potential radicals or troublemakers. As a new nurse you must focus on your nursing skills and on figuring out the strengths or weaknesses to the social rules of your department, as well as identify your friends and foes before you can ease into a comfortable position.

Nurses require many interactions with patients, their families, supervisors and administrators with each interaction *or scenario* being different. A nurse should be in a care giving protective role when working with patients, in the role of equal when working with fellow nurses, and in the role of subordinate when interacting with administrators and supervisors. The varieties of nurses' social interactions all require different interpersonal skills thus making affiliation complex.

Conclusion

This chapter has exposed you to the social structure of a medical institution. Make sure you learn and respect the people at the top of the ladder. Find a comfortable level of interaction within the social structure. The most important factor for success is working for a fair charge nurse and your relationship with him/her.

Learn to value and evaluate the many kinds of interactions. Most interactions will be valuable and helpful but learn to discriminate. You will work better in a hospital where nurses cooperate and collaborate. In order to collaborate well with coworkers you have to have the same beliefs and the same likes and dislikes. As the new person you will have to be open to change, eager to learn, and able to see beyond your own private opinions and beliefs.

Remember to use caution when dealing with nurses who give assistance. You have to make sure your relationship stays as informal assistance rather then formal supervision. Also when dealing with nurses who give advice, if you comply all the time you run the risk of reinforcing bossiness and being told what to do more often. Choose carefully which nurses to obey and try to find out which nurses go to the supervisor if their suggestions are not carried out. You don't need any more bosses so don't create any. You learned you will need a support group in any healthcare situation. Even with a diverse staff you can build an adequate support system. The suggestions in this chapter have helped you learn to deal with getting this support. Also remember there are friends and then there are friends at work. You need friends at work but now you realize in what context and to what extent.

The nurse can solve affiliation problems that involve relationships with patients, families, fellow nurses, and administrators. It is important to seek solutions to these problems because the quality of interactions and the degree of affiliation with others greatly affect feelings of personal and professional satisfaction.

You now have a better understanding of the social order of a hospital. Being a nurse is being smack in the middle of this social order. The rules, hints and procedures outlined in this chapter will help you with these social order relationships and you will find you can ease into any nursing situation.

Chapter 5

Meet The Nurses

This is the chapter that will tell you about nurses' personalities and their lives. I assume you wouldn't be reading this unless you were interested in knowing what a nurse's personality was all about. Here is the chapter that's going to answer that question for you. Then you can decide what you want to do with it.

The hospital being discussed could be any hospital, certainly any hospital in a big city or surrounding area. In fact it could be almost any hospital in the country except for a very small rural one. Hopefully you did your homework and the hospital that you are starting to work in meets your criteria.

There are many stereotypes of nurses. They are depicted as angels of mercy, mother figures, handmaidens, and sex symbols. Is this what nurses are really like? Are there nurses who weep for their patients, fight the odds of their alcoholism or drug addition, defy doctors who treat them badly, cope with corporate business people and save lives? Some of the people you might find yourself working with will probably make up a colorful crew, normal but colorful. They will be people who dedicate their lives to nursing and caring for people.

Something Special to Offer Nurse

There is Margaret. She is the nurse that can work with terminally ill patients and can give them something special. She is a middle-aged woman with short blond hair and has the hint of a European accent when she talks. She seems to be a real city person. She has two grown children and has been married since she was twenty. Since nursing school she knew she wanted to give something special to dying patients.

When you watch her work you see she talks to her patients on their level. Right now she is working in a children's cancer care unit. She will tell the children and their parents what will happen and how the drugs will work in a way that they can understand. She administers all the chemotherapeutic drugs and stays with the child to the end, whether the end is a cure and life, or death.

She likes working with the child and the parents early in the disease. That way they learn how to deal with the psychosocial implications as well as how to deal with the effects of the drugs. She makes sure parents know how a disease will change their child's life and how it will change the family and how to manage so it isn't devastating. She helps the child understand the disease so it doesn't become overwhelming and distort their life. That's how she gives them something special.

The children and the parents became very dependent on her; they will call her when they need answers. There was David who was born with congenital leukemia. He'd been disease free for several years. Then at six his symptoms returned. It was devastating to the family. The physician was matter of fact about the course of chemotherapy and other procedures. It didn't help David or the family very much.

David knew he had a serious illness and might die. He opened up and talked to Margaret about it. He drew pictures and was able to tell her his fears. His mother and Margaret became very close. They would talk, Margaret would give her the factual information but even more she would listen and comfort her. When David died, his mother told Margaret she would never have been able to get through it if it hadn't been for her help and support. They still correspond even though it's been several years since David's death.

The Mother Figure

Mindy is a soft-spoken, warm compassionate woman. She is single with no children of her own. She has been working for a County Hospital for twenty years and worked herself up through the ranks in the hospital. She now works the night shift on the Psych floor. There aren't any doctors around at night and if patients are lonely, they have no family to comfort them during those hours.

These patients have both mental and physical problems. Mindy helps them get in touch with their feelings. She talks with them so they understand the effects of what is happening. Many patients will complain of lower back pain or abdominal pains and she finds that rape, incest or other types of physical abuse are the underlying problems. Mindy will use imagery to relax the patients. She will tell them to imagine a peaceful scene. Sometimes all she can do is hold a patient's hand. To her that is what a nurse is there for, to comfort and give human touch. She feels when she has a patient who is suffering terribly what they really want most is someone there to touch them and be with them.

One of Mindy's patients was a drug addict who had been raped. She said she started using drugs because of the rape. She complained of excruciating abdominal pain. She supposedly was off drugs. Everyone felt the patient was just imagining the pain. After Mindy got to know the patient she decided that the pain couldn't be imaginary because of what she had observed and learned about the patient. They gave her all kinds of tests and finally found the cause of the problem and were able to alleviate it through medication. Mindy feels each of her patients is her responsibility, like they were her children. She gets to know them in a way no other medical person on the case does. She will make it her business to find out what the patient really needs.

Ethical Value Nurse

Nurse Maria was an extremely religious person. She believed in preserving life at all costs. She was a woman in her late twenties, married with three children and one on the way. She was hired as a temporary relief nurse to come in and relieve a man who was caring for his terminally ill wife. He hadn't been out of the house in several weeks. The wife was terminally ill and didn't want to be on any life support if and when the time came. The doctors orders stated do not resuscitate.

Unfortunately the wife stopped breathing when Maria was on duty. Maria wanted to start resuscitation procedures but obeyed the doctor's orders and did not. The husband was extremely upset when he found out his wife had died. Marie felt she had gone against her own belief in not resuscitating the women and felt the women could have lived.

Maria didn't impose her ethical values on a dying, suffering patient but she felt a great deal of pain because of this. She followed the doctor's orders. As a nurse you must learn to let patients and their families do things their own way. When you first become a nurse you may think you know what is best for the patient regardless of their wishes. This usually causes a lot of pain and anguish for the patient and their families, especially if you do not have the same ethical values. A nurses' personal value system should not get in the way of the patient's own wishes for their care.

Personal Integrity Nurse

Joe has been a prison nurse for ten years. He is a very liberal man one who doesn't judge people. He just sees people as either needing nursing care of not. He also likes to live a little dangerously and likes to make his own decisions and be in control of his work. Prison nursing seemed to give him the freedom to be the type of nurse he wanted to be. He faced the dangers of caring for murderers, rapists, child molester and drug dealers day after day. It tested the limits of his commitment and his integrity but he loved it.

His day begins at five AM with the prisoners' count. After that, he tests the diabetics and draws up their insulin. Then he gives tranquilizers to the inmates who need them checking to be sure that inmates don't hoard the pills. He doesn't have enough help to do all the checking. Tranquilizers are given in liquid so inmates can't hoard pills and overdose. In the morning he usually has a lot of patients with colds, fevers, etc. Most of them are not serious. Joe gets a little frustrated when he has a real emergency like an asthmatic attack, and an inmate who wants attention for a stuffed nose both at the same time. Some inmates consider sick call a sort of social time and Joe has to limit their visits to twice daily.

He has to handle a lot of substance abuse cases and psychiatric problems. He feels his goal is not to completely cure or rehabilitate inmates but to make them social enough to be integrated back into prison life. With the limited medical services available to him, he feels he is lucky if he gets them well enough to participate in prison living and court hearings. Ninety percent of the prisoners have some type of addiction. They really don't want to kick their drug and alcohol addiction. In jail they are forced to withdraw because they can't get anything. Medically speaking Joe takes what steps are necessary to get them through it.

One of the things that surprises new nurses who work with prisoners is that prisoners don't recognize their alcoholism and drug addiction as a problem. They see their lifestyle as every bit as legitimate as yours or mine. If a new nurse works with prisoners thinking, "I'll help them kick their habits and have a better life" she is going to be sadly disappointed.

Joe has revulsion toward crime but he still wants to provide care to the criminal. Most of the time he doesn't even know why the person is in prison. He knows he doesn't have the power to reform anyone. He accepts that the prisoners mostly do not want to be reformed or even admit they have a problem lifestyle. Joe has learned to care for the people without judging them. Some nurses can achieve this in their careers and others can't. You have to decide what kind of nurse you want to be.

The Military Nurse

Andrea has been an army nurse for thirty years. She came from a large family and decided to join the Army Student Nurse Corps in order to finance her education and maybe even see some other parts of the world. She really didn't like the idea of joining the army, she wanted to be freer than what the army would allow but she had no other viable plan.

After graduation she worked in a series of positions and in a few years volunteered to serve in the Gulf War. She was curious about what was going on at the front and wanted to see how she could help the critically wounded. She was made charge nurse at the front, and worked fourteen to sixteen hours a day. There weren't many physicians, she learned to make quick assessments and institute procedures with or without a physician's orders. She did this in order to save lives.

At night she covered all the units herself. If a patient had an emergency she would handle it. She often took on the physicians' role and the corpsmen assumed the nurses' duties. Her patients really respected her. She got to know her patients, she became like a mother or sister to them. They'd tell her about their experiences in the field. They would reveal their fears of the war to her. She became very attached to them and tried to never let them down.

The enemy had no respect for the hospital or the wounded and she found herself in many scary situations putting her own life on the line. The enemy would plant bombs on roads or there would be sniper fire right in the camp. The hospital where she worked was built close to the airstrip and ammo dump. This caused the enemy to try to bomb the location that the hospital was in. The working conditions were like slum conditions. She was able to cope with it physiologically but some nurse's couldn't and had nervous breakdowns and had to be sent home.

Nothing could have prepared her for what she saw and had to do. Either she was going to be able to handle it mentally and physically or she wasn't. If you decide to become a military nurse take these issues into consideration. It is not an easy job. You may find yourself away from everything you know in hostile, almost unbearable conditions handling patients like a physician. It could stretch your mental and physical capacities to the limit and challenge every one of your beliefs and abilities.

The Inner City School Nurse

Ann is a school nurse for approximately fifteen hundred children. Among the students there are learning disabled, emotionally disturbed, and high risks children. She also runs a clinic where she does health risk screening, physical assessments and lifestyle counseling. She is an attractive woman in her forties with two grown children.

Her job has changed drastically in the past few years. Drug abuse has doubled, children as young as ten can be dealing drugs. The surrounding neighborhood has become more dangerous, funding for programs have been cut, and truancy is up. There is little respect for the healthcare worker and she had to become quite street wise in order to survive.

She feels she never has enough time to handle all the emergencies that come up. She administers daily medication to the prescriptive students. She handles all the emergencies. She finds lunchtime is the most dangerous time. There are emergencies daily during lunch hours. The worst situation is when a child has to be taken to the hospital and their parent or guardian can't be located. In those situations she goes to the hospital with the child. Ann has learned to cope with the overcrowded conditions and the inconsistent information on health records.

The neighborhood can be dangerous at times. Ann found out which places are safe to go into and which are not. Once she let her guard down, while going to her car and didn't look around to see if there were any suspicious people around. When she got to her car a gang of boys closed in on her. Luckily people at the school saw what was happening and started yelling and the kids dispersed. Ann wasn't hurt but it took its emotional toll on her. It was a couple of weeks before she was able to walk to her car alone.

Ann is now a very streetwise non-judgmental person. Like Joe, the prison nurse, she has learned to work under unsafe, unorganized, and unreliable conditions. She has learned to accept the culture of the population in the school where she works. She never pushes her own beliefs on her students. She is there to help them mentally and physically. If you decide to become a school nurse and find yourself working for an inner city school you will have to embrace this type of attitude in order to fit in and help your students. Each school is different and the bigger the school the more varied the situation becomes.

Nursing and Substance Abuse

Nurses like to deny that they are vulnerable to addictive behavior such as alcohol and drugs. But this is a problem in the medical profession. Sara is a woman in her late thirties. She has a quiet beauty and most patients want her to be their nurse. She is a recovering alcoholic. She had

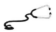

denied she was an alcoholic for a long time. Nobody at work suspected she was drinking she never missed work and seemed to function.

Her husband was a physician and worked long hours. He did what many other physicians did to keep up the hectic pace. He took sleeping pills for insomnia and stimulants to keep him up. At the time neither one saw anything wrong with his drug abuse. This was partially due to Sara's own addiction to alcohol and partially due to the fact that it was common practice in the health field. Eventually her husband was put in the hospital. She became depressed and began drinking again. She just didn't care. She was almost suicidal. Somehow she managed to call the Women's Crisis Line and ultimately admitted herself to an alcoholic unit.

Before this happened she felt she could handle everything herself. She never confided in others. Now she has partners in AA who she calls anytime of the day or night for help. Sara is back at work under supervision. Her urine is tested and she receives counseling. She does service work by counseling hospital nurses on substance abuse, but doesn't tell them her own story.

Most people do not understand how this could happen to a doctor or nurse. Doctors and nurses think that alcoholism and drug addiction will never happen to them, and they can't tolerate it when it happens to their colleagues. Some nurses imply that they succumb because of the stress of their jobs. Others say it's because the person had a predisposition to it. Substance abuse is something that can and does happen to the healthcare professional. Just become aware of the dangers and take precautions to protect yourself.

Conclusion

These are some of the personalities of nurses you might find in any health facility. Most nurses exhibit some form of personality traits described in this chapter. In every hospital there will be the, Something Special Nurse, who can give that special something to dying patients. There will always be the, Mother Figure Nurse who treats her patients like they were her own children. Then there is the Ethical Nurse who feels she knows what is best for her patients even if it is not what the patients want.

The Personal Integrity Nurse is able to treat any type of patient and not judge them.

This chapter also made you aware of the possibilities and dangers of substance abuse in the medical profession.

If you are just starting out in your nursing career, give yourself a few weeks and you will be able to categorize most of the nurses. You can learn from each nurse's personality. Pick out the good traits of each nurse and model yourself after him or her. Key in on what personality traits are not working and avoid falling into the same traps. Find what personality traits work best in what situation and pattern yourself from that. Most nurses are within the normal personality range and will be helpful to you. One or two might be dangerous to your job. Use each personality to your best advantage and find the best traits to help you ease into a health facility. Select a unit where you have the best chance of being treated fairly. Try to work in an institution that has similar beliefs as your own. The other nurses in your unit are one of your most important resources, so use them wisely.

Chapter 6

Patients and Their Families

A nurse can establish a relationship with patients and family that can create magic in the healing process. Nurses have knowledge apart from medicine. They treat human responses to health problems as well. The nurse evaluates how the patient and his or her family are adapting to the social and psychological effects of the illness. Her reactions and method of helping can and does have a great influence on the recovery of the patient.

The essence of nursing is to interact and invest time and knowledge in other people's lives in order to heal. The nurse's investment in other people's lives is not without a price. Most patients and their families welcome the helpful nurse but some may reject her well-meaning efforts, or test her. How the nurse responds to the patient's needs, will depend on her level of education, experience, commitment and the time afforded her to do her nursing. The majority of real nursing is self-monitoring, assessing, guiding, teaching, nurturing, supporting and counseling patients and their families.

Patient care is a constant responsibility for the nurse. The nurse should become sensitive to the patient's mental as well as physical changes. An unspoken word, a cry of pain, a cough, uneaten food, a change in color of surgical dressings all can trigger the nurse's senses to a change in the patient's healing process. The nurse registers these systems and decides what action should be taken if any. Her presence over time allows the patient and family to form a relationship with her. The patient and family may disclose things to her that they would not with anyone else.

No other profession challenges your values and ethics like the medical profession. You will enter the nursing profession with your own set of values that have been developed by your religious and cultural environment. As a nurse you will have to learn to override your own personal beliefs for the benefit of the patients, their families and the facility where you work.

Your own beliefs will have to be put on the back burner in order to coexist with patients their families and the facility where you work. You may feel life should be maintained no matter what. But maybe your patients don't feel that way. Or maybe that's not the main attitude of your colleagues or where you work. You will have to learn to bend your ideals in order to comply with the wishes of the patients, their families and the beliefs of the facility. No one wants to tell you this but if you want to succeed as a nurse this is what you have to learn to do.

As a nurse, your beliefs and attitudes are a major concern in every day decision-making. The way you handle your beliefs verses that of the patient their families and the facility will determine if your succeed as a nurse. The patient's wishes should always come before your own unless it's against the law. You should become attuned to the attitude of the department that you work in. Your colleagues are a great source of information for this.

Constructive Relationship With The Family

It is very important that you form a positive relationship with the patient's family. You will find you need to work with some families more than others. Dying patient and their families will be more in need of your help then most others. Try not to impose your personal beliefs on them but instead listen to their wishes and help them carry them out. You also might find yourself caught in the middle knowing more than you are allowed to tell them about their illness.

You will have to find the best spot between the families, patients and the hospital. Should nurses assume family roles when the family can't manage? Can the nurse instill respect for the healthcare treatment if the family discounts its worth? The family and their home environment also influence a patient's recovery. Are these influences more important than the treatment? The patients create this environment in part because their illness is the product of their family and life. Patients and their illness are better addressed when you have family cooperation. By drawing family into the patient's treatment you can better address the issues and healing of the patient.

Nurses know that home and family affect a patient's progress and illness. When the family and home life are positive, the patients will usually heal faster. If the patient comes from an unstable family where he has little support, it may affect his healing in a negative way. Although there are exceptions to the rule there seems to be a connection between the patient's family and the healing process. Patterns of family visits and connection to the treatment of the patients will mirror your patient's progress.

As a nurse you will want to have close collaboration with families. Sometimes you will get satisfaction from your work just because you didn't get any family complaints. Some nurses feel intimidated by strong families and others like and seek the families out. Either way will work, and you will find which works best for you. Nurses and families are on the same side in that they both want to do what is best for a particular patient. Therefore if you look at families as allies, then you can establish communication. As a nurse you cannot expect your professional authority to go unquestioned, for sometimes families will question your nursing skills and you will have to be able to defend yourself.

There are many different types of families. There are families who can make a nurses' life miserable for the whole time she takes care of the patient, by constant phone calls and question about the treatment. There are some families who believe by virtue of having to pay the hospital bill that they can expect nurses to serve as the patient's private caregiver. Then there are the families that are most grateful to the nurse for whatever she does.

Despite the difficulty that nurses sometimes feel when confronted by an occasionally intrusive family member it is less worrisome than the habitually absent one. Most nurses want and seek family involvement for their patients even if not for themselves. There are many factors that promote or inhibit participation in the patients care. Unquestionably, some family members' life circumstances, wealth, work, health, or family obligation influence the extent of their involvement and the patterns of involvement.

How To Talk To Families

Some helpful hints for success when talking to families:
Check the names and relation to the patient of all involved.
Be cordial in your greeting.
Answer all questions about the treatment in an honest and positive way.
Never give information that only the physician should reveal .
Try not to take comments personally.
Listen carefully and let them participate.
Present the positive and the negative, but start with the positive.
Be sensitive to the nonverbal.
Call the attending physician if need arises.
Never be negative about the patient's progress .

Quality Nursing

Some nurses exhibit quality behavior that cannot be measured. For instance if a patient is comatose some nurses will focus on the family. What place does the family want in the person's dying? Do they want to be with him? Talk to him? Some people can do this very easily, while others can't.

There was a comatose patient, Harry, and when his wife entered the room he became more alert and when the nurse said, "Harry, your wife is here hold her hand", he actually put out his hand for her to hold. His wife was happy that some progress was made in his illness. She became very friendly with the nurse and a bond was formed between them to get Harry better.

Terminal cases need a lot of attention from the nurse and their families. The nurse can be the catalyst who brings the family closer together for the patient's last days. There was a patient we'll call Jane. She had cancer and it spread to her bones, which made it quite painful. She loved to go out to dinner. The nurse and her family wanted to help her do the things she loved to do. The nurse went to her home at dinnertime and with her help the families was able to all take her out to dinner. They had to be careful moving her and had to give her a lot of pain medication but she was able to go. They all worked together to enable Jane to do the things she thought she would never do again.

Families That Can't Cope

Sometimes there are families that can't cope with the illness, or resent the illness and what it is doing to their family. Other families can't emotionally take care of the patients. Or maybe the insurance ran out and the family had to pay the bill or take care of the patient themselves. They may call the nurse all times of the day.

One woman had a little girl with liver problems; She would take the child back and forth every day for her hospital treatments. She had a younger child at home and a husband who separated himself from the sick child. He couldn't bear the sorrow of seeing his child dieing. He couldn't emotionally support the mother or the child. But the mother felt this was her baby and she was going to do whatever she could to keep her alive. The nurse tried to prepare the mother for the inevitable death of the child. The nurse spoke to the mother and gave her as much support as possible. A bond was formed and the mother didn't feel as isolated and alone. When the little girl died, the nurse comforted the mother. If the nurse weren't there the mother would have had no support.

Another case is a fifteen-year-old schizophrenic boy, David. He was hearing voices and wasn't able to function. During the boy's stay in the hospital his parents came for a family group therapy session. During this meeting, family members including David discussed the transition from hospital back to the home. David's father was very upset with David and blamed him for his illness. He felt the boy could stop hearing voices if he wanted to and could be like other kids. He felt David could be normal if he really wanted to. Underneath the father was really scared. David understood he had a chronic illness that he could control if he took medication and continued therapy. But the father couldn't understand this.

Families who Keep Information From Patient

Sometimes, family members may want to conceal information from the patient as well as other family members, such as children. They may feel it would be too stressful for the patient or other members of the family if they knew everything. This can be perceived in two different ways, one way is that people who keep information from the patient or others do so because they themselves can't accept it. This may be so in some cases but more likely it is an act of love. Either way this can be a difficult situation.

The main problem with this is the people who are excluded do not have a chance to get to resolve what is happening. They may guess what is happening but decide it is not what they are allowed to talk about. You may have to deal with the person who wants to keep the secret in order to help the patient and the whole family. You do not want to be caught in the middle of this. In most cases it is best to try to get the secret out and get the family communicating

The strategy that works best is to negotiate with the secret holder and get him or her to talk to the other family members. You can find out what the family members and patient knows. If the patient knows or has worked out what is going on then the problem is solved. The benefits of attempting to break the secret is that the family can then talk to each other and begin to sort out their relationships and life and how best to cope with the situation.

Family Solution is in Conflict With Patient's

A problem may occur if a family's course of action is in conflict with a patient or the health professional. If several solutions are voiced then the person who has the problem, most likely the patient should get his way, provided that it is practical to do so.

One area where there is much family intervention is in the care of the elderly. Many older people living on their own want to be independent but their family members may feel they are not able to any longer. In these situations the family often overrides the solution that has been worked out by the elderly member.

As a nurse in these situations your main goal is to assess the situation and prioritize the problems. Encourage the patient to generate their own solutions, set realistic goals based on the best options from the patient's perspective and help evaluate the outcome. As a nurse you can offer to listen and to help them find their own best solution. You and the patient must also accept that occasionally there is no easy way out of a particular situation.

Family Controlling The Dying Patient

There was a bachelor who was terminal ill with cancer. He was in excruciating pain. He didn't speak up for himself because he was too sick. He couldn't even get out of bed himself. His sisters came and forcefully took him back to their house. They took away his identity. They decided on what kind of treatment he should have even if it was against his wishes. It was true he hadn't been taking care of himself in the best way but it was the way he wanted too. He loved looking at the mountains and wanted to die by the mountains. When they took him to their home he was no longer able to see or be near the mountains. He died the way his sister's wanted him to, not the way he wanted to.

Other commonly heard stories involve strong willed adult children who control how their parent will die. One mother hid her illness from her high society daughter. Finally she could hide her pain no longer. The daughter insisted she get medical attention and when she did it was diagnosed as inoperable cancer. The nurse made house calls and gave the mother the care she needed. The mother was on medication but didn't seem to want too much else. A conflict began between the daughter and the mother about her treatment. The nurse became squeezed between the mother and daughter's wishes.

The nurse began to conspire with the mother against the daughter rather then fight the strong daughter. Finally the mother couldn't fight the daughter any longer and surrendered to the daughter's wishes about her treatment. When this happened the mother's condition got progressively worse quickly and she died very soon after.

As a nurse you will learn the value of letting patients do things their way, especially in terminal cases. At first you may think you know what is best for the patient, just like the daughter thought she knew what was best for her mother, and the sisters who thought they knew what was best for their brother. In the end they just denied the person the right to die as they choose and with their own dignity.

Nurses Who Speak Up For Their Patients

Unfortunately, many hospitals don't know how to handle some patient's pain. The nurse has to become aware of a change in a patient's discomfort level and call a doctor to get the help needed for the patient. As a nurse you have to learn to get help for your patients.

One evening, a cancer patient in a city hospital became confused and combative. The staff thought the confusion was a reaction to methadone and stopped giving it to him. Now he was in terrible pain and just moaned and moaned. The family didn't know what to do and begged the nurses to do something. One nurse gave him Demerol and Vistaril but that hardly had any effect. The wife was beside herself because she couldn't bear seeing her husband in so much pain. She begged the staff to do something. One nurse did, she called the doctor even though it was in the middle of the night and a morphine drip was started. This nurse spoke up for her patient even though it was against hospital procedures.

Families That Blame Themselves

Inherited diseases can be a source of guilt for the family.

Especially in child cases of inherited disease the family is more prone to blame themselves for the child's illness. Parents and grandparents may blame themselves for passing on the disease to the child. Or they may blame the other side of the family for the inherited disease. In these instances the nurse should help the family to understand that blaming isn't helpful to anyone, especially the patient.

Don't Take It Personally

It requires a great amount of diplomatic skills to handle patients and their families day in a day out. You have many personalities and cultures you must deal with. If you have done everything you can and all fails don't take it personally. An example of this is, a new nurse had an older woman patient who was dying. They had just transferred her to ICU to the oncology floor and the family wanted to get morphine into her very fast, and on a regular basis. The family either couldn't stand her suffering or had other reasons. They told the nurse they did not want to prolong the women's suffering. There was some nastiness among the family members that gave the nurse a funny feeling. The nurse was waiting for the pharmacy to enter the orders since it was a transfer and had to be processed. It was a very busy night and the pharmacy was very busy. The family demanded immediate service. The nurse called the pharmacy several times to get the morphine. While she was doing this the family called the charge nurse, and the nursing supervisor to complain. The nurse was working as fast as she could but she had no control over the pharmacy. She wasn't working fast enough for the family.

The nursing supervisor of the whole hospital came to speak to the nurse. The supervisor told the nurse the family was extremely unhappy with the care given and it was unacceptable and she wanted to know what had happened. The nurse gave a little laugh partly out of anxiety and partly out of disbelief. She had done her best , the waiting time for the medication was out of her control. The laugh was perceived as an attitude and she was told, "That is what the family is talking about," they had said she had been judging them. In that instance, the supervisor was actually siding with the family. The nurse was taken off the case, she felt betrayed and outraged. But she decided not to take it personally. She had done everything she could. It had been out of her control. You must learn to not take some things personally.

Conclusion

Each patient and their family handle illness in their own way. Some are comfortable in sharing their pain, while others are not. Most families need temporary help to get them through the illness. The nurse is there to guide them in developing skills needed to cope. As a nurse you will find out very quickly that it is important to have a constructive relationship with the patient's family. If you want to succeed in nursing this is what you must be able to do.

This chapter has given you insight into not putting your own beliefs ahead of the wishes of the patient and their families. This chapter explored the different types of families and how to handle them. It gave examples of families that blame themselves, families that control the dying patient, and families that can't cope. It gave you hints on how to help and guide these families through these trying times. As a nurse you will need these skills to succeed.

It also helped you understand what to do when you are caught in the middle of knowing more then you are allowed to tell the family and patient as well as other situations. As a nurse you will find yourself in these kinds of situations regularly and now you have the strategies to deal with them successfully. You will have learned when to use your influence and when to put your job on the line to benefit the patient. One way to find out what to do in these situations is to look to your colleagues. Observe what the experienced nurses do on the floor. When do they call the physician on behalf of the patient?

This chapter taught you how to deal with all types of families. It has provided you with helpful hints for dealing with any family situation. The guidelines in this chapter have shown you how to successfully deal with patients and their families in order to benefit all involved.

Notes

Janet Kraegel, R.N., Mary Kachoyeanos, R.N., "Just A Nurse", (E.P.Dutton 1998)

Suzanne Gordon, "Life Support", (Little Brown and Company,1997)

Echo Heron, "Tending Lives, Nurses on the Medical Front", (The Ballantine Publishing Group, 1998)

4.   Ann Faulkner, "Effective Interaction with Patients", (Churchill Livingstone 1998)

Chapter 7

Meetings

There are many different types of meetings in the healthcare profession. The type of facility where you work will determine the type and frequency of meetings you will have as a nurse. You may have large staff meetings if you work in a hospital or small patient/ family meeting if you work in home care. Interviewing and assessing the patient is an important factor in nursing. Whatever the situation meetings are an essential part of your job as a nurse. You must learn how to make meetings work for you. This chapter will enable you to do this.

Staff Meetings

Staff meetings are usually part of a large hospital's agenda. They are informative and will help you learn what you need to know to take care of the patients on your floor. Usually the charge nurse leads the staff meetings. As a new nurse the best thing to do, at any meeting, is listen carefully and follow what is suggested. If you don't understand something ask another nurse after the meeting. Try not to say too much or ask to many questions during the meeting. You don't want to look like you think you know it all by saying too much and you don't want to look like you are incompetent by asking too many questions. Try to stay within a happy medium.

A Sample staff Meeting

A registered nurse, Ann, usually works evening shifts, but today she comes in early for a staff meeting. It has been four days since she worked. At the meeting she is filled in on the patients conditions. She finds out the patient, Ellen is very bad. She is failing and afraid she will die. Another patient, Dee, died during the morning shift. Her son couldn't believe she was dead until the mortician came. He had tried to get the nurses to start an IV.

Lucy a cool professional nurse, who knows how to keep her emotional distance, reports on the patients conditions in matter of fact way, "Mr. Jones' ulcer is worse today", she exclaims. "Try to change his position every two hours tonight. Miss Waves is going to the general hospital in the morning for a biopsy." She pauses, insinuating saying at last, and then continues. "Mr. Comer has refused to eat again today. Maybe it's time for a feeding tube or psyche consult. I wrote his doctor a note. Jim Moor needed morphine twice on the day shift. He seems to be getting worse. The morphine barely holds him for four hours. His doctor is probably afraid he will get addicted. Poor guy probably doesn't have another month to live. I wish we could make him more comfortable. Everyone else on the floor is stable."

The meeting continues with the night nurse speaking about her favorite patient, Sara who died last night. She found her already blue and stiff. She felt ashamed, guilty and sad that she was not with Sara when she died. Every death reminds her of every other death she's ever seen. Now she wants to record this event while the details are vivid in her mind. The way her skin changed, the way her eyes seemed empty. She wanted passionately to remember her patient.

The chaplain takes over the meeting and the nurses talk about the emotions they take home from work. The chaplain emphasizes that the public sees healthcare professionals as dedicated people whose aim is to help the sick. In reality nurses are human beings who hurt like any other human being, and caring for sick patients year after year can take it's toll on one emotionally.

There are many ways a nurse can cope with emotional burnout.

You may have to emotionally distance yourself from the patients. Find the right amount of professional involvement, which protects you emotional. Try to communicate with the patients as completely as possible but in a professional way. The more you communicate with patients and their relatives, the closer you will get to helping the patient and also achieving your own peaceful emotional state.

Interviewing the Patient

Today patients have more input into their own care, and if you want to succeed as a nurse it's important that you sit down and listen to them. A lot of the time a patient will reveal something important to the nurse that they would be uncomfortable telling the doctor. You can learn how to anticipate a patient's concerns.

The assessment interview with the patient will set the scene for planning appropriate care for the patient. Some important factors while interviewing a patient are, where and when to have the interview, privacy and time allotted. The right time is when the patient feels comfortable talking. The amount of time is relative to how the time is used.

Whether you are interviewing the patient at home, in a clinic or hospital, privacy is important. A private environment can help the patient disclose problems and concerns that are needed for assessment. As a nurse you will not have ideal conditions when planning an interview. Many wards do not have private rooms where a patient can be interviewed. People in there own homes often cannot locate an area where they can be alone with the nurse. Telephones ring, Do Not Disturb signs go unnoticed, children rush in and occasionally a partner tries to insist on remaining present when the patient is assessed.

All you can do is try to find a quiet room where the patient will feel comfortable and there will be as much privacy as possible. Try to make arrangements to divert phone calls. Put, "Do Not Disturb", signs up and explain to the people around that you do not wish to be disturbed. Sometimes in hospitals the best that can be achieved is the illusion of privacy. In the patient's home you may have to ask for the TV to be turned off, the phone to be taken off the hook and to be undisturbed. The best insurance is to always make an appointment and mention your request for privacy.

Review Available Information

After the time and place of the interview have been set, you should find out what information is available about the patient. Notes, and letters of referral both help to paint the picture of a patient's background, history, and current condition. Some patients feel comfortable when a nurse who is interviewing them actually knows something about them. Such foreknowledge shows you had interest in the patient and his problems and took the time to get their background information. Some difficulties in knowing the patient's background on the first interview is that it might cause you to make prejudgments and maybe miss new factors.

Background information can be useful as long as it is used constructively. Retain the information but ask the patient to tell his story in his own words. This will give you a clear picture of the patient's understanding of what is happening to him and show you any mismatches between what the patient believes and his history.

When interviewing patients, use open-ended questions, questions that cannot be answered with simple, "Yes" or, "no" responses. A nurse may ask "Can you tell me how this all started?" This is a good example of an open-ended question. It gives control to the patient. Open-ended questions allow the patient to express their feelings. "How did you feel when you found the lump?" In open questioning you don't assume anything about the patient's perception of his illness.

You will also have to facilitate during the interview, meaning you will have to try to overcome obstacles and make it easier for the patient to verbalize concerns. Try acknowledging the patient s problems and then show your willingness to share. The other things that help facilitate disclosure are empathy and educated guesses.

Empathy is the ability to feel what the other person is feeling. It is hard to feel what another person feels especially if your own experiences have not been part of theirs. It is possible to build a picture from an individual's interview so that you can begin to understand their reactions and feelings. Try to imagine what they are going through.

Educated guesses help make for understanding hypothesis. You can use all the collected information to make an overall assessment of the patient's situation.

Also check whether other interviews have taken place recently or if one is scheduled in the near future. If for example, a long medical interview has recently taken place then you, as a nurse may want to postpone your interview. You do not want the patient to feel overwhelmed with questions. It is also important to explain the nature of the interview. This helps the patient understand that everybody is not repeating the same task.

Some steps in dealing with patient interviews are:
Find the best possible quiet uninterrupted place where the patient will be comfortable for the interview
Give yourself enough time for the interview
Make whatever arrangements necessary for an uninterrupted interview
Review background information
Identify physical, psychological and social problems
Determine the patient's main concerns?
Explain who you are and the reason for the interview
Check to see when other interviews have or will occur
Ask mostly open-ended questions.
Use facilitation, empathy and educated guesses in your questioning

Cues, Diversions and Maintaining Focus

An interview should be patient led. In order to do this you must be able to key in on cues given by the patient. Patients do not give cues one at a time or in order of importance. You may be given a number of cues all together and then you have to sort them into their order of importance. If you ask the patient to identify their most important concern and then offer to discuss it with them, you will start the interview in a structured and focused way.

The priority that the patient gives to certain concerns may not match what you think are most important. This can be a problem for you. It might be tempting to focus on cues that have to do with the patient's physical problems primarily because these may be easier to deal with than social or psychological problems. Try to key in on the cues that the patient is most concerned with and try to deal with them first.

Patients may find it easier to divert talking about the things that are bothering them. If you allow this to happen the concerns of the patient can get lost completely. An effective diversion controlled interview may be very painful but it will allow you to know the patient and his needs. You can handle diversion by acknowledging it and then going back to the patient and their problems. Do not allow the patient to talk about other things. Acknowledge the other things briefly and then go back to the patient and their needs.

Keeping focus during an interview means being able to negotiate, control the conversation in a caring manner and to acknowledge difficulties. Try to stay focused on the patient and their concerns. Some patients will have difficulty staying focused on a painful subject. If a patient cannot talk about a particular painful issue you should note it and try to bring it up again in the interview.

Assumptions and Beliefs

Try not to make assumptions during the interview. There are common problems associated with any illness and it can be tempting to assume your patient has these problems. A self-fulfilling prophecy may result in that a patient may feel they should have these problems even if they don't if during the interview you assume they do.

What a patient believes about his illness is as important as what he knows at a logical level. By finding out the patient's beliefs it is possible to understand his responses and solutions to his illness. For example there are many misconceptions about cancer. By letting the patient tell his beliefs it is possible to understand his misperceptions and then you will have some chance of correcting them.

Become aware of your nonverbal skills. A verbal, empathetic

response needs to be linked with appropriate behavior if the message is to be believed. In general if the verbal and the nonverbal messages do not match then the nonverbal message is the one more likely to be believed. If you ask the patient, "Tell me how you feel?" you must then be prepared to wait and hear how he feels. If your non-verbal signals suggest that you are not interested then the patient will realize this.

Exploring Feelings

During the interview, patients will not only describe facts about their situation but they will also describe their feelings. Patients might be reluctant to express their feelings even when you make it clear it is all right to do so. They may feel their worries are trivial. You should encourage a balance between the expression and exploration of feelings. Once feelings are expressed that give you a clear picture of the patient's main concern then you have to try to help the patient find a solution or comfort zone. To do this you must be in control of the interview in a sensitive and helpful way.

Talking in itself can't solve problems but it can be therapeutic in helping to put problems into their proper perspectives. When problems are discussed the impossible situations can be put into a manageable solutions.

Screen and make sure you have a clear picture of the patient's feelings. Acknowledge what you don't have control over and move on to something you can control. Not every issue can have a happy ending. The help you can give by interacting effectively is to assist the patient, to clarify his or her feelings and begin to move on to possible solutions to current solvable problems.

By helping the patient explore his feelings it is possible to get a picture of how likely he is to accept new information which may necessitate a change in lifestyle that may help his condition. Information should be given in a way that the patient can understand. It is hard to accept that sometimes giving information to a patient even when fully understood does not mean they will comply. A diabetic may understand how to treat his condition but he may not adapt it to his own lifestyle and decide not to stay on a restricted diet. Some patients may not comply with information given them because it is too drastic a lifestyle change. An example of this is smoking. A patient may understand perfectly that smoking is affecting his health but he may decide to continue to smoke.

Giving Information to the Patient

Meetings with patients give them the opportunity to discuss their worries and concerns. Many patients' concerns come from lack of knowledge about their illness. They may not know how they can take care of themselves. During the interview it is essential to give information that you feel a patient should have and also the information the patient requests. Patients are often anxious and confused when they first enter a hospital. The anxious patient is less likely to understand information. Information should be given to the patient in a way they feel comfortable with. Use language they understand and in the proper social context. The average person can take in about seven pieces of information at any one time. The anxious patient probably less.

Since the Access to Medical Records Act 1988, patients have been allowed to see their own records on request. Studies have shown that most people want as much information about their illness as possible. Let the patient lead you in knowing how much information he can handle. Give information in meaningful chunks, stopping when the patient has had enough or is satisfied that his questions are answered. Try not to say anything that is opposite of the doctor or hospital recommendations.

Some rules on giving information to a patient are:
Identify the patient's current knowledge.
Give the information you feel he should have and what he requests.
Decide on a plan, with the patient in the lead, to improve their knowledge and care of their illness.
Assess the patient's understanding of the information
How did the effect of the information leave the patient feeling

Typical Interview

Mary is a hospice nurse. She sees three of four patients each day. First she reviews the background information then calls and sets up her one-hour appointments. She begins by reminding them of her privacy needs and gives the reason for her interview. She starts her interviews with an open question such as, "How has it been since I was here last" She then listens, validates and assesses their concerns. She keeps careful control over diversion techniques, while using empathy and educated guesses. She addresses any problems that are within her control to help the patient reach solutions. She keeps in mind that patient concerns are the most important, even if they do not agree with hers. She will arranges for an expert to come in if she can't handle a problem herself.

She uses a team approach. The team usually consists of the nurse, medical social worker, physician, home health aide, homemaker and or volunteer and chaplain. An assessment of the patient is done and Mary makes sure she answers all of the patient's and family's questions. Then she summarizes the visit to make sure everyone understands what he or she needs to do with the care and process.

Assessing the Interview

If you conducted an effective interview you would have had gathered information about the patient and his problems. You will have gained insight into the patient's reaction to his problems and related emotional issues. It is hard to accept that what might seem to be the major problem to you might not be most important to the patient. If the patient's main problem is an emotional one then that is what should be addressed. You should encourage the patient to set priorities. Then you must negotiate with respect to what can be solved and managed by the patient. When your priorities are different from the patient's and you feel it is essential to tell them, make sure you present them in a way that they are equally important and for very cogent reasons.

The hardest part of identifying the patient's problems is having to accept their decisions, which may not be the best solution to the problem. The patient may refuse a blood transfusion because of religious reasons.

On an emotional level the patient might remain in an abusive marriage. Knowing the logical solution doesn't necessarily mean the patient will accept it. The patient should generate his/her own solutions whenever possible in order to have the most success. Interviews need to be conducted so that care can be planned on the basis of the patient's perception of his problems, rather than on what we think his problems are.

Conclusion

Whatever the situation, meetings are an essential part of your job as a nurse. In order to succeed you must make meetings work for you. This chapter has given you the information in order to do this. Many different types of meetings were discussed such as types of staff meetings, family patient meetings, and how to interview a patient. Suggestions were given as to how to conduct yourself for best results with sample meetings and rules being provided.

Issues during a patient interview such as privacy, the right time to have the interview and the time allotted for it, review of available patient information, cues, diversions and maintaining focus, assumptions and beliefs, feelings, as well as when and how much information to give a patient were discussed in this chapter. Steps and rules were given on how to deal with the many issues that may arise during an interview and how to best handle any situation.

Helpful hints were also given on how to conduct yourself during any type of staff meetings. The sample meeting provided a realistic view of what to expect at a typical staff meeting. Staff members will work successfully together if they all value communication with each other and the patients. At individual and group supervision sessions and meetings, nursing care plans should be discussed and pulled together as a team would. With the helpful suggestions provided in this chapter you will be able to make any meeting work for you.

Notes

1. Cortney Davis, Judy Schaefer, "Between the Heartbeats", (University of Ohio Press,   1995)

2.   Ann Faulkner, "Effective Interaction with Patients", (Churchill Livingstone 1998)

3.   Jane Schweitzer, R.N., M.P.A., "Tears and Rage". (Adam-Blake Publishing,1996)

Chapter 8

Patients and How to Protect Yourself

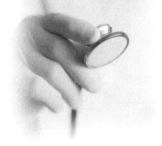

What the Nurse Likes

I like looking into patients' ears
And seeing what they can never see
It's like owning them
I like patients' honesty-
They trust me with simple things:
They wake at night and count heartbeats
They search for lumps
I am also afraid

I like the way women look at me
And feel safe
Then I lean across them
And they smell my perfume.

I like the way men become shy.
Even angry men bow their heads
When they are naked

I like lifting a woman's hair
To place stethoscope to skin,
The way everyone breathes differently
The way men make suggestive groans
When I listen to their hearts

I like eccentric patients:
Old women who wear purple knit hats
And black eyeliner, Men
Who put makeup over their age spots

I like talking about patients
As if they aren't real, calling them
"the fracture" or "the hysterectomy"
It makes illness seem trivial

I like saying
You shouldn't smoke!
You must have this test!

I like that patients don't always
Do what I say

I like the way we stop the blood,
Pump the lungs, turn hearts off and on with electricity.
I don't like when it's over
And I realize
I know nothing

I like being the one to give bad news,
I am not embarrassed by grief.

I like the way patients gather their hearts,
Their bones, their arms and legs

That has spun away momentarily
At the end of the gathering they sigh
And look up

I like how dying patients become beautiful.
Their eyes concentrate light. Their skin
Becomes thin and delicate as fog.
Nothing matters anymore
But sheets, pain, a radio, the time of day

I like watching patients die.
First they are living,
Then something comes up from within
And moves from them
They become vacant and yet
Their bodies are heavy
And sink into the sheets.

I like how emptiness is seen first
In the eyes, then in the hands

I like taking care of patients
And I like forgetting them,
Going home and sitting on my porch
While they stand away from me
Talking among themselves.

I like how they look back
When I turn their way

By Cortney Davis

Patients, you have to love them in order to care for them. Then the love has to change into tough love, because you must put your emotional feelings aside in order to help them within the guidelines that the institution gives you. You may know what would really help them, but if the doctor doesn't prescribe it, or if the institution doesn't provide it, or the patient doesn't want it, you simply cannot do it. You have to harden up and face the fact that you are not going to help every patient the way you know how; rather, you are going to help the patient in the best way the institution, your job description and the decisions the patients makes allows. Both you and the patient will have to conform to the doctors, institution and family wishes. The patients who are supposed to get better will, maybe not in the fastest way or the best way, but they will get better. Don't try to save the whole world; just try to save a little bit of it at a time.

Caring For Patients

The nurse has a specific role in the care of patients. There is something wrong if you cannot connect to a suffering human being: but you also must keep a safe emotional distance. Patient relationships with nurses can become complicated. Caring for patients entails more then just physical care. You have to mentally care for them as well. Some patients need more care then others and some will affect you more emotionally than others. Not only are you caring for them physically you are caring for them mentally also. How they react to you is a major part in their recovery. Patients affect your mental health and you affect their mental and physical health. This is a great responsibility and you will have to learn how to handle and protect yourself from certain situations with patients.

When you care for patients realize that you have to abide by their wishes, their families wishes, their physicians' wishes and the facilities wishes. As a nurse you will get intensely involved in some of your patient's lives for a short time. During this time they may become very dependent on you. Even during this dependency time you will not have much to say in any major decisions making. You will have to learn to handle yourself by abiding by the decision of the patient, their family, their physician and the hospital.

When a person goes to a doctor with a problem, the doctor diagnoses it, suggests a course of treatment and believes that treatment is the best available at the time. If anything goes wrong the doctor might have to defend that treatment. As a nurse you will have to take responsibility in the same way. You may have to defend whatever care you give even if the patient gave his consent for that treatment. Most appropriate decisions are made when there is good negotiation and understanding between patient and health professional.

The most difficult times are when a patient or family member asks for inappropriate treatment such as in terminal cases. The family may want the patient to be force-fed or a drip put in a dying patient. You must carefully assess the real motive behind these unrealistic requests. Often the person is seeking a miracle. Try to get them to talk about their real feelings and maybe they will acknowledge the reality of the situation.

The patient and his family do not have to accept the suggested treatment. You may find it hard when a patient does not decide on the best solution. An example may be a patient who is overweight, a smoker and a heavy drinker who just had a heart attack but doesn't want to change his life style even after good reason was given to him. If the patient makes the informed choice to continue this life style you will have to accept it. Your main aims are to encourage the patient to find his own solutions based on information he has been given. You can suggest solutions based on the doctors and medical facility procedures. What needs to be clarified is that the patient who makes the decision takes the responsibility for doing so and doesn't come back and blame you if something goes wrong.

Avoid giving the patient a solution yourself. Guide the patient into finding his own comfortable solution. You should only offer a solution when a patient has exhausted all his ideas and found none to be acceptable. Then proceed with caution. Sometimes a solution may have to involve the family. A problem may arise when a family's solution is different than the patient's. Try not to get in the middle between the patient and the family even if you strongly agree with one verses the other. You don't want to be the referee or the mediator. Let the patient and family find their own comfortable solution.

A patient may have a problem that is beyond your control to help. For example clinical anxiety or depression may need psychiatric help. You must follow the procedures in these instances. Referring another doctor will not be effective without the consent of the patient. You may have to redefine the patient's definition of the help you are suggesting to him. An example would be explaining why and how a psychiatrist would help. If the patient then refuses to see anyone it is his right but you have done your job. But to fail to do this could have caused a problem for you.

Types of Patients

There are many different types of patients just like there are many different types of nurses and doctors. Everyone handles sickness differently. Some people quietly accept it while others become aggressive. Some express guilt, denial, fear, depression, or have spiritual issues. Severity of the illness and length of time in the hospital can also determine how the patient behaves. Patient's personalities basically stay the same. If they are an optimist they will remain optimistic. If they always found a cloud in every silver lining they won't suddenly at age seventy-five see the world through rose colored glasses.

The patient's psychological state is a great determining factor in their progress. Many things can contribute to the patient's mental state such as family, friends, their physician, type of illness, knowledge of the prognosis, control or lack of control of medical decisions and general attitude toward getting well. Included in this, is the nurse's reaction to the patient. The nurse is the first person the patient and their families ask questions of. As a nurse you will have to know how to answer these questions in a positive manner without lying or overriding the physicians or hospital's polices.

Some hints in doing this are:
Find out what the patient already knows
Explain the treatment in a understandable manner
Always be positive
Stick to what the doctor ordered
Don't say anything against the hospital's policy

Each patient has different needs and motivational drives. A nurse may find that sitting by one patient in the middle of the night is all that's needed while another may need constant talking for consoling. As a nurse you can't expect to change a patient's behavior. You will have to become attuned to their needs and try to fulfill them while staying within the guidelines of your job description.

The Angry Patient

It is common for patients to feel angry in response to an illness. People look for a reason for things that happen in their life and when they can't find one they become angry. An example of this is a man who lived a healthy life, never smoked, exercised regularly, and ate a healthy low fat diet but he got a heart attack. He felt he had lived a good healthy life so why should he get a heart attack. He also felt he was a good husband but his wife was leaving him. He can't find the reasons for his situation so he becomes angry.

When dealing with the angry patient it is important to acknowledge the anger, make it legitimate and allow the patient to vent it. Only then will the anger begin to dissipate. If you ignore it or try to rationalize what has happened the anger might get worse.

Some steps to follow in dealing with an angry patient are:
Acknowledge the anger.
Find the cause.
Encourage positive expression of anger.
Attempt to defuse it by encouraging positive solution.

All the while you must stay within the boundaries of the doctor and hospital policies. The focus of the anger may be inappropriate. You may have a patient who is directing his anger at some aspect of his care or at you personally. Even a relative of the patient can become angry. This can happen particularly after a patients death. A relative can come to the ward and get angry with you. It is important in these situations to not be defensive. Locate the underlying cause and the real focus of anger and then try to defuse it. Once the focus of the anger is identified then thoughts can be shared and the anger defused. The first question you should ask in a situation like this is, " I can see how angry and upset you are. I wonder if we can talk about this for awhile". Also, add into the conversation that you know it is hard for them to understand the death of their loved one but you really don't believe they feel all this anger toward you. Try to find out who or what their anger is really at.

Guilt

Many patients feel guilty; the patient who has lung cancer who smoked may feel guilty. Parents may believe they caused their child illness and feel guilty. Bereaved family members sometimes have guilt feelings. Most individuals wish they had done more for the person that died. Sometimes guilt is perfectly justified but sometimes it is without foundation.

It is not possible to take guilt away but talking about it makes it possible to put the guilt in its proper perspective so that people will have some chance of forgiving themselves. You can deal with the guilty person, whether it's a patient or family member, by acknowledging the guilt and then trying to put it in it's proper perspective. What you can't do is take the guilt away with reassurance or absolution. You may want to try to get the person to look at it in a different way and ask if perhaps he is being too hard on himself. If guilt feelings are not identified they may grow out of proportion and the individuals involved may need to get psychiatric help before they can come to terms with it.

Denial

Denial is not uncommon with patients that have a serious disease. It can happen to relatives who do not want to accept the reality of what is happening to a loved one. It occurs when a situation is so difficult that the person has to put it out of his mind as if it does not exist. The difficulty with denial is it become hard to talk about the situation thus affecting the treatment and solution.

The strategy you should use in dealing with denial is to find out first if they are in complete denial or whether there is some ambivalence. That is, one day he may acknowledge his illness and the next day not. If the individual can accept some reality than there is some hope in helping. You should understand that some patients need denial in order to cope, however you should not feed it. Use natural responses such as, "Well I hope you will be well enough to do that." instead of, "I'm sure you will be well enough to do that". This more neutral approach does not break the denial but if the denial is replaced with reality the patient will not feel that you have deceived him. So trust between you and the patient will be maintained.

Fear

It is natural for a person when faced with an illness to be fearful. The fear may be about the effect of the illness, the treatment or the relationships or other social aspects. Some may fear their families will stop caring for them if they are not perfect. It is important for you to identify whether their fear is within normal range. If you talk to the patient about what is frightening him this allows the patient to put the fear into context. The reality of being in a hospital and being under care may take away the fear because the experience may not be as fearful as anticipated.

You can help the patient overcome their fear by facing it with them and discussing it. Whatever their fear is they must find the solution. You can only talk it over with them and help them find a comfortable way of solving it. If the fear is at a level where it is having negative effects and is interfering with normal coping mechanisms, it may be necessary to refer them to expert help.

Depression

It is typical for a patient to become depressed, particularly if his disease is life threatening or will bring permanent change to his life. If depression is identified and treated the patient should be able to move on to address the problems that has effected his emotional state. If depression continues and is severe it will require psychiatric intervention. You may have to discuss this with the patient's doctor if you find the patient in an uncontrolled state of depression.

Spiritual Issues

There are many different types of spiritual beliefs. A patient may want to talk to a religious person or he may want to ask you an existential question. Questions are usually put to a person they trust. The difficulty is when you don't know the answer or if there is no one answer. In handling spiritual questions you don't have to know the answers you just have to be willing to listen and discuss issues that the patient may be struggling with. It is best not to get involved in religious beliefs so refer them to a minister, etc.

Listen to their spiritual concerns without trivializing them. The most common theme is the loss of control in the illness situation. By helping identify their concerns you can help them begin to find solutions.

Dealing With Patient's Death

Being a nurse requires boundaries. As a nurse your responsibilities are to enable your patients to get the best out of life physically and emotionally. Once their spirit leaves this life there is a line which you don't cross. Feeling pain over a patient's death is inevitable when you connect with them and see them as more than a disease process or a chart. One of the responsibilities in nursing is being able to share in the human experience, of which death is a large part.

The only problem comes when your response to a patient's deaths overwhelms your normal functioning in some way. Then I would consider seeking help. With spiritual and emotional maturity, you will be able to share in this experience without becoming overly distressed.

It never gets easy to lose a patient. Since we don't hold the key to life, it's not our choice. A greater power sometimes lets us win and keep our patients and sometimes no matter how hard we try the power takes them away.

There are some people who can have a positive outlook on losing a patient. You can try to assess the situation and rationalize that the pain and suffering the patient is experiencing can only be relieved by death. You are not losing a patient the patient is gaining relief. It can be a wonderful experience to help someone cross over from this life to the next. It doesn't always have to be a terrible thing. You can feel lucky to have been a part of the patient's life at the end by spending quality time with them and their families. Some nurses rely on the fact that their patients are no longer suffering and death is seen as a relief. These will be times when you will hug the family members and cry with them. As long as you can cry you are working in the right place

Nurses are taught to be healers, but not every patient is going to go home well. We do not hold the keys to that kingdom. You can't take the pain of grief away. We all have to go through that emotion so that we can heal, and if we allow that to happen it can make us a more compassionate and caring person.

You also have the choice to respond in a cold and unfeeling way by shutting your own emotions down. If you do this, you will be loosing a lot. There is much to be learned from the dying client. The patients you will remember most are the ones that make the most impact on your life during the last few days of their lives. Ask them questions about how they are feeling if they are able to tell you. What are their most important memories. What would they do differently. What advice would they give you. You can be given greater truths about life by getting answers from these types of patients. You will find rewards when you can see beyond the pain. You will fondly remember certain patients that made an impact on you and realize that person changed you in some way. That person lives on because you now carry on a part of that legacy. Strive to be the kind of nurse that you would want to take care of you.

At every passing you may feel a piece of you has left with them, but remember a piece of them stays with you too. Each of us is different and what might be good for one might not work for you, so find your outlet. Talk with someone you're close with at work. Each experience will represent something different in your life and will give you great rewards.

One of the hardest things to learn as a new nurse is what to take seriously. In the beginning you will not always know what subtle changes signal an emergency. Here is a story about a new nurse's plight. This first year nurse Jane, was in charge of a psychotic women patient in her eighties with advance kidney failure. On the day she died the family called the hospital and asked Jane if she thought the woman was going to die. Since Jane observed the women looking good she told the family she was stable but a few hours later the woman died. Jane felt awful. Some co-workers told her that patients often look better before they die. But if Jane had told the family that the patient was near death they could have come to the hospital to pay their final respects. Nowadays, Jane avoids the trap of predicting death, she simply says, "We have no way of knowing when someone is going to die".

Number of Patients

One of the major problems in nursing is the number of patients in your care. The unit and severity of patient illness is a factor in the number of patients you can safely care for. You can have a one to one in recovery and a 12 to one on a floor. Four patients per nurse are ideal for a general floor. Twelve patients with assistance can be the norm in some hospitals. Again you will have to learn to conform to the policy on patient load depending on where you work. Do your homework find out what your patient ratio will be before you accept the position.

Laws and Your Rights

Your rights as a nurse will vary depending on what state you work in. A OB-GYN nurse working in FL may be able to screen all her patients for AIDS but a nurse in Boston will find she needs legal consent from the patient. This can be a problem. You should know whom you are dealing with but the law doesn't grant you this privileged.
It is the nurse's responsibility to know the laws of her state and the policies of the hospital.

By law, every patient is to be treated equally, they are entitled to the same health care. Whether they have insurance or not, whether they are criminals or saints, whether they are famous or not, you are supposed to administer the same level of care. The motto being, "Exceptional Care without Exception". Any experienced nurse can tell you that there are patients and then there are important patients. You will probably be asked to give special treatment to certain patients for whatever the reason. They could be celebrities or relatives of influential people. Whatever the reason just go along with it and give the special treatment when asked. It will make life a whole lot easier for everyone involved including yourself. You don't want to get on the bad side of a supervisor because you wouldn't help out with a special patient. No one wants to tell you this but this is what you have to do to survive in the nursing profession.

How Much Do You Tell A Patient

It is always hard to know how much to tell a patient. If you tell them too little they will blame you for not telling them enough, if it becomes necessary for more treatment. If you tell them too much they may become overly concerned and become frightened. You can ask your colleagues for help when you are not sure how much you should tell a patient.

An example of this is a man in his fifties who was admitted to the hospital with chest pain. His doctor told him if the pain continued he would need a cardiac catheterization and possibly open heart surgery. Obviously, the patient did not want to admit to the pain. The nurse on duty knew he was ignoring his pain. The nurse spoke to him and convinced him that if he told her when he was having pain it would be better for him. Once he admitted to the pain they decided to do a catheterization. After the procedure he was told he had a blockage in an artery and they wanted to do an angioplasty but didn't think it would work and he would need a by-pass. It was very upsetting. The nurse didn't want to add to his anxiety but she felt he needed to know what to expect if he needed surgery. The man was upset with the nurse. He felt everything got worse because he told her about his pain. He mistrusted her now. The nurse understood his mistrust but she told him what to expect if he needed surgery. (You will need to get MD approval for this.)

You will have to make decision as to how much, when and what to tell a patient. Look to your colleagues for help in this matter. Find out when and what they tell patients. It might depend on which doctor the patient has as to how much you can tell them. Or it might be the hospital or the department polices which will determine the safe amount of information you can give to a patient. Either way as a new nurse your colleagues will be the best models for you.

Listen To The Patient

There is a fine line between a patient knowing what is best for themselves and the doctor's diagnosis. As a nurse you don't want to get caught in between. An example of this is a doctor who tells a nurse that a pregnant patient is not ready for delivery. The patient says she feels she is. The doctor leaves. No sooner is he gone than the woman starts to deliver her baby. When the doctor returned the woman had delivered in the labor room. The doctor then became mad at the nurse and wanted to know why she hadn't brought the patient to the delivery room.

The patient stood up for the nurse and told the doctor he had said she wasn't ready and it wasn't the nurse's fault. This was good for the nurse. If the patient hadn't stood up for her she could have found herself in a situation with the doctor and the patient. From then on this nurse took careful consideration when a mother to be said she was ready to deliver her baby. Depending on the type of patient you have to decide whether their input is valid.

> Some questions to ask yourself in deciding are:
>   Is this the type of patient that can have insight into his own diagnosis?
>   Is his illness the type he can have insight into?
>   Is this patient knowledgeable about his illness?
>   Does this patient deny his symptoms?
>   Has the patient been through this before, ie. childbirth?

It is important to include patients in the decision making process about healthcare. Healthcare should be a team approach. That team should include the nurse, physician and most importantly the patient. Nurses can help patients be involved by educating them about their medical needs and diagnoses, helping them understand. It's important for nurses to make sure patients have appropriate information so they can be informed decision makers.

Many patients are very well informed because of greater access to clinical information through the Internet, the library, etc. Still, nurses are needed to help patients integrate outside information with specifics about their own personal condition.

> As a nurse you can help the patients by:
>   Making sure all their questions are answered.
>   Making sure they have a list of their medications.
>   Making sure they get test results.
>   Making sure they understood the procedures their doctor recommend.
>   Making sure they understand what will happen to them if they need surgery (with MD approval of course).

These steps can help a patient understand that they aren't passive recipients but should be involved in decision making. Involved patients and families as well as nurses can help reduce medical errors and improve quality care.

Bending The Rules For Patients

You will find that bending the rules with some patients will help both you and them.   There was a patient, Jack who fell into this category. He was a patient you talked about over coffee because he was so demanding and he was a heavy smoker. He was a patient who was more challenging than most.

Toward the end of the first day Jack started to go through nicotine withdrawal. He asked for a cigarette about ten AM. The hospital's policy and all the dangers of smoking were explained to him. He seemed a little convinced. He was given a Valium. By eleven AM. Jack started to get aggressive. He wanted to be unhooked from the heart monitor and allowed to walk down the hall for a cigarette. One cigarette that's all he wanted.

The nurse just couldn't unhook him from the heart monitor, he was told that she was responsible for him, and off the monitor his heart rhythm couldn't be watched. He grabbed the intravenous tubing and screamed, "I'll pull this goddamn thing out, you watch me" He was really yelling and pulling at his hair. The nurse decided it was time to call the doctor.

When the nurse explained the state Jack was in the doctor rationalized that if Jack discharged himself from the hospital he would go home and smoke himself to death. So they decided to let him have three or four cigarettes a day just to keep him sane. They decided that everyone would take turns walking Jack down the hall with a portable monitor, and praying he didn't have chest pains while having his cigarette. He would time his cigarettes to the minute and he could make it on four a day.

This seemed to work out well for everyone. The patient was content and stayed in the hospital where he could be monitored. The nurse was able to do her job. The rules were bent but with a positive outcome. The nurse did get consenting okay from the physician so she was not alone when she broke the hospital rules. There seemed to be good reason and good outcome for breaking the rules. So bending the rules were done in a positive way that benefited everyone.

How to Protect Yourself Emotionally

Patients recover and go home, others get worse and linger, while still others die. In every situation, as a nurse you will become emotionally involved. To what extent depends on your personality, relationship with the patient, type of patient, how long you were caring for the patient, and the diagnosis. If you work in a children's transplant unit you may become more involved than if you work on a general floor. You have to know how much you can get involved in a certain patient's life without it having ill effects on your own. As a nurse you have to learn how to protect yourself emotionally because it can become too much to handle if you don't.

Obviously, if the patient gets better and goes home this is the best outcome emotionally for everyone. Some patients linger, get worse and die. You have to be able to handle this emotionally. You will have to find the best way emotionally for yourself. Find the right unit for your amount of emotional strength. You can't cure everyone but you can make it easier for the patients as they are dying and for yourself.

Sometimes a patient's problems become too close to your own for you to help them find their comfortable solution. For example, you may have a patient who is in an abusive marriage and maybe you had a similar experience and find it too painful to say nothing. You may be at risk of using your own experience to persuade your patient in finding their solution. The patient may become too dependent on you and blame you if something goes wrong. In situations like these you should ask to be relieved of the patient.

Everyone has his or her own way of dealing with the emotional stress of a job. Become aware of signs of loss of enthusiasm, positive attitude, confidence , self-esteem, and depression within yourself. Try to find your limit in the emotional involvement with your patients.

Some techniques that can help you adjust to the emotional strings of nursing are, don't take your work home. Consider hobbies, relaxation time, humor, professional group participation and talking. Something as simple as changing your clothes when you get home form work may make it possible for you to cut off work emotionally. Find the ritual that helps you forget about work when you are not there. Any hobby can take your mind off the emotions you will experience at work. Find something you enjoy and do it. Give yourself relaxation time to be pampered. Get your nails done, have a message, whatever it takes to make you feel special. Find the humor in any situation and find the good things in your day. This will help you cope with the emotional situations. Join a professional group. Sometimes just talking to someone about your feelings will help you put them into their proper place.

One of the most important paths to emotional good health is to work in a supportive environment. Find other nurses that you can collaborate with and want to become your support group. (See chapter 2, Support Groups) They will probably be the nurses on your floor. Talk to them, ask their opinions, express your feelings and ideas.

Conclusion

As a nurse you must learn how to deal with many different types of relationships with patients. The most important issue discussed in this chapter is the realization that you may know the best solution for the patient but if the doctor doesn't prescribe it or if the institution doesn't provide it or if the patient or family don't want it, you simply cannot do it. The best solution is the one the patients make for themselves and it may not coincide with yours. It was revealed that your main aim is to encourage the patient to find his own solution based on information that has been given.

Types of patients, such as the angry, guilty, in denial, fearful, or depressed patient were discussed, as was the best ways of dealing with these issues. Different ways of dealing with a patient's death, spiritual issues, how much to tell a patient, when to listen to a patient, and when to bend the rules for a patient are also stated in this chapter.

You must learn how to protect yourself when dealing with your patients. The helpful suggestions suggested in this chapter such as, don't take work home with you, hobbies, relaxation time, humor, professional group participation and talking will enable you to do this.

Notes

1. Ann Faulkner, "Effective Interaction with patients", (Churchill Livingstone 1998)

Chapter 9

Complaining

As a new person you will be evaluating and comparing the procedures and methods used at the facility where you work. You will have your own ideas as to how things should be done. At times you will want to express these ideas. There is a way of doing this in order to achieve the best results. You will want to learn how to express your ideas so that you do not alienate anyone, especially your supervisors, or you will seem like a know it all who is now telling everyone the right way to do things.

Expressing you ideas can be viewed as a form of complaining. There are basically two forms of complaining: constructive complaining and unconstructive complaining. Constructive complaining is when you know how and to whom to complain to bring about positive results. Unconstructive complaining is complaining done in the wrong way, and to the wrong person thus causing more harm then good. There will be times when you are tempted to complain, but before you do, make sure you have done your research and know the constructive way to complain for positive results. Have a plan, know whom to go to and have the answer or a better alternative prepared in advance.

Learn to complain constructively. Complain only to the people who can really help. Make sure you complain to the right person in the right way at the right time. Find out the proper protocol for complaining in your facility. Is the best protocol to go straight to the head of the department, or do you go to the charge nurse, or the union representative with constructive complaints first. Find the right person. Find the best time to talk to this person and in what way. Do you have to make the complaint sound like something else or can you talk straight to this person? So do your research, find out which ways work best with which people. Also find out the relationship people have within the facility. You don't want to make the mistake and complain about the charge nurse's cousin because you didn't do your homework.

Unconstructive complaining will only hurt you mentally, physically, socially and financially. If you complain in an unconstructive way, you might get a bad name. No one likes to listen to a constant unproductive complainer. You may make enemies who see you as a new member who feels everything is not being done her way. When you first get into a facility you have to be cautious about complaining.

Supervisors are willing to help and listen to complaints, as long as it doesn't make their job harder or longer. The supervisors hired you to do a job, not to make their job harder or longer. Be cautious when complaining to the supervisors; make sure your complaints are not going to make their job harder. As a newcomer you should keep complaining to a minimum.

Constructive Complaining

Healthcare is a stressful world, a medication error can be fatal, a patient can take a turn for the worse with no warning. Sometimes little gratitude is expressed and criticism is the rule rather then the exception. Complaining is an easy way to get anger and aggression out rather then face the situation head on. Those with lower self-esteem may use complaining the most. They may try to feel better about themselves at the expense of their colleagues, and work conditions. Complaints that start off as professional gripes sometimes end up as personal attacks. You must learn to use complaining constructively. You want complaining to work for you, not against you.

You will find that the nurse's lounge will become the group therapy room. Complaining can provide group unity when a universal target such as a disliked doctor or hospital policy is agreed upon. Battle stories can be shared in an atmosphere of camaraderie among those similarly wronged. Complaining does have its part in easing into nursing, you just have to learn how to complain in a constructive manner.

Learning how to complain constructively is a very important component in the nursing profession. Some hospitals bring in assertiveness trainers to teach nurses how to channel their anger constructively.

Ten steps to constructive complaining are:
Make sure complaining will accomplish good results.
Complain to the right person.
Find out how to complain properly to that person..
Find out the proper protocol from your colleagues.
Do research on people's relationships and programs before complaining.
Don't complain about any nurse who has been there a long time.
Don't complain if it's going to make the supervisors work harder.
New nurses must keep complaining to a minimum.
Don't complain when you are angry.
Don't constantly complain to co-workers.

Doctors and Nurses Relationships

If at all possible don't argue with the doctors. As a new nurse you will always lose. Nurses are not seen as equals to doctors. Most doctors will treat you with the professional respect you deserve but unfortunately some feel nurses are there for their convenience to blame or criticize. Sexual harassment can also be a part of the doctor – nurse situations. It is difficult working with these types of doctors. Some nurses handle these insults with passive acceptance and indirect expressions of anger. Others want to take some form of action. Most frequently the emotions felt are fear, anger, anxiety and frustration.

Verbal and nonverbal outbursts by doctors have to be handled carefully and tactfully. Going one on one with a doctor will probable only make a bad situation worse. If the patient is in jeopardy, unfortunately the best way to handle it might be silence. There will be time to resolve it after the crises. If you antagonize the doctor further by criticizing him in front of the patient it will very likely make it worse for the patient and yourself. This is hard for a new nurse to understand but this is one of the dark secrets of the healthcare system that no one wants to tell you but you should know if you want to succeed in the profession. The doctor can and will go to your senior staff nurse (charge nurse) and complain about you. They will probably side with him and you will be reprimanded. This is not the way to ease into any nursing position.

Sometimes, standing up to the doctor by explaining why you weren't able to do something to their liking might help. An example is: A doctor berated a nurse for not answering the phone quick enough. She explained that she was assisting another physician with a procedure on an elderly patient and with all the equipment running she didn't hear the phone. Some doctors can be reasoned with by giving an explanation.

In other situations such as sexual harassment you may not feel comfortable confronting the physician. You may want to ask the department supervisor to do so for you. You may prefer to send the doctor a letter, with copies going to immediate supervisors and the chief of medical staff. Again be very careful before doing this. Putting something in writing should be a last resort. Find out from your coworkers and union representative if this is the best way to proceed.

Nurse doctor relationships are improving because of nurse's education today. Many nurses are graduating from colleges with Bachelor degrees. Many go on to get Masters and Doctorates. Physicians with 8-10 years of education are now working with nurses who have 4-9 years of education rather then three years of nursing school. The handmaidens of the past are being replaced by the specialty trained. Nurses are starting to demand the respect that goes with highly educated individuals and doctors are beginning to comply.

In most hospitals especially in large teaching hospitals this relationship of doctor and subordinate nurse has changed. Today there are many female doctors. Many of these new doctors liked to be called by their first names and are bringing new levels to their relationships with nurses. Still the main emphasis is on complying with the doctor's wishes whenever possible. If you want to ease into a position you will have to learn how to work congenially with the doctors as well as standing up for yourself. Complaining about them or to them is not going to help you much.

Nurses Relationships

Relationships among nurses in a facility should be healthy, congenial, cooperative, friendly, and interdependent. You must strive to achieve healthy working relationships. Friendly cordial talk in lounges about families, movies, or weekend plans will help develop healthy relationships. You need to be part of the group in order to ease into the department.

Some behavior that might help achieve this relationship is to talk about nursing with your colleagues. Observe and share each other's ideas. Work together on patient's care; learn from each other. A healthy work environment is characterized by good relationships among the staff. You have to change your thinking from, "I" to "we" in order to accomplish a relationship with your fellow worker. Think in terms of, "All of us will work together, help one another, and make our knowledge available. We will work collaboratively for the benefit of everyone.

Within any staff there are norms and groups. It is helpful to understand this informal staff organization when trying to understand nurses relationships with each other. There are a number of bases for staff groups, including age, family background, attitudes, seniority, and common interests and activities. Most nurses belong to overlapping groups. Different groups have different degrees of prestige and authority within the facility. Entrance into the top group is gained by having recognized competence that is highly valued by the charge nurse or department head.

To become a member of a group involves identifying group expectations and then trying to meet them. Presented next is a self evaluation questionnaire. The items on the self-evaluation questionnaire represent some of the more common practices that can help your relationships with other nurses. As you answer, think about whether each statement reflects an expectation you hold for your colleagues. After you finished, evaluate your answers. Note where you may need to work on your relationships. Try to put yourself on the receiving side of these statements with other nurses. Would you like these things done to you? How would they affect your relationship with other nurses?

> Do I criticize or report fellow nurses to the charge nurse?
> Am I considerate of my colleagues?
> Do I gossip about other nurses?
> Do I interfere in other nurse's work?
> Do I complain about my duties?
> Do I engage in petty arguments?
> Do I criticize any previous nurses' achievement with a patient?
> Am I sympathetic to other nurses' problems?
> Am I jealous of other nurses' successes?
> Do I expect things to be done my way?
> Am I constantly talking about how things should be done?
> Do I belittle my co-workers or charge nurse?
> Do I settle complaints in a professional manner?
> Do I go to the charge nurse with petty problems?
> Do I spread rumors?

Optimism

Be optimistic. How successful you become could depend in part on your general outlook on life. Those who generally expect good things to happen are more likely then less-optimistic people to achieve their goals. An optimist will try to overcome obstacles when confronted with impediments to goal attainment, whereas pessimists are more likely to cease striving because pessimists have less favorable views about how things will turn out. Complaining can be a form of pessimistic behavior.

You may find that looking for ways to demonstrate your positive belief in others will help you ease your way into nursing. Negativity is one of the great weapons of management and administrators. By keeping nurses divided between shifts, units, new hires and experienced staff, etc. managers create an impotent, fractured workforce. When infighting is present administrators have less to worry about because nurses who are divided don't unite to fight for better working conditions. It is rare that a manager prefers their staff to be divided but it does exist. Most managers will want their team to work together.

Consider your own general outlook. Do you believe that most situations will turn out in your favor? Do you strive to produce desired results before circumstances get out of hand? If you cannot answer these questions positively, you might try substituting positive forecasts for those in which you predict bad outcomes. Planning ahead is also a useful tactic. Further, acting in a more enthusiastic manner, greeting others with a smile, and keeping a list of all the good things that happen could lead to greater optimism. Most nurses can benefit by avoiding the habit of describing their circumstances negatively.

Nurses do hold expectations for their colleagues, and many nurses are concerned about how others view them. A nurse's experience in her first position or any new department situation contributes to a firmly developed view of herself as a nurse. Yet any new nurses entering a department, will find that worker relationships are fairly well formed. As a newcomer, you will find yourself at the bottom of the order, an outsider in relation to the department and its culture. You will have to discover and accept the norms and procedures of the department. You will have to make an effort to fit in. You will have to mold yourself to ease in and be accepted.

Needs of Nurses

Nurses are all individuals with very different needs, and those needs affect expectations. If you are a new nurse and a young adult you might be occupied with selecting a mate, learning to live with a marriage partner, starting a family, rearing children, managing a home, getting started in a profession, taking on active civic role, and finding a congenial social group. In contrast a new nurse in mid life, having accomplished these tasks to some extent, is confronted with a different array of needs. She may be interested in achieving adult civic and social responsibility, establishing and maintaining an economic standard of living, assisting teenage children to become responsible and happy adults, developing adult leisure time activities, relating oneself to one's spouse as a person, accepting and adjusting to psychological changes of middle age, and adjusting to aging parents. The differing needs of these two groups could naturally lead to different expectations for professional experiences.

Needs of individuals cannot be stereotyped by merely describing age groups, but it is critical to remember that personal needs alter professional expectations and affect interactions with others. Recognizing this fact requires your being sensitive to others and trying to understand other's points of view.

Outside Interests

Many nurses report that having interests outside of healthcare facilitates, develop and maintain total well being. Balance in work, health, social, and leisure activities are essential to personal and professional growth and development. The impact of too much or too little attention in any area can spill over and produce negative consequences in the other areas. The person who works day and night on healthcare assignments can destroy their family life or other important relationships. The nurse who relies solely on work for a sense of personal worth may act resentfully toward colleagues who fail to be equally committed to the pursuit of healthcare. In fact, any negative experience on the job could have far reaching impact because the job is that person's whole life.

No exact formula is available regarding the amount of time one should devote to work versus outside pursuits. What is required for a healthy balance will vary from person to person. You must find your happy balance by trial and error. If you find that work related activities are interfering with you family life to a stressful degree then this is a clue that you are devoting too much energy to work related activities.

Affirming the worth of others will include listening to others, looking for their positive qualities, responding positively to others, and considering the frustrations of others. Listening is a procedure that all nurses can use to improve their relationships with others. Listening is helpful because it permits nurses to learn more about what others think and feel. It also communicates the nurse's concern for others, which in turn makes others more receptive. Effective listeners get actively involved in what others say and they demonstrate empathy for the speaker. Becoming actively involved in what others are saying often begins by recognizing that you have something in common with them.

People tend to get into a certain acceptance routine. They have learned to accept and maybe not even notice those things that will be blatantly obvious to you as a newcomer. You will wonder why these obvious things are not complained about by any of the people that have been there for awhile. You will soon find out that there is a good reason why no one seems to notice them. It's because if you notice and complain, you will get into more trouble than it is worth. Some things in a hospital are not debatable; so no one mentions them.

For example, you may notice that certain people really don't do their jobs properly. Maybe the nurse's aid whose job it is to take certain patients down to x-ray doesn't do this in a timely fashion. When you did your research you soon found out why. She was part of the "inner circle" of the charge nurse's friends. She had been at the hospital longer then anyone and knows many of the higher ups when they first started there. Everyone had grown accustomed to her habits. If anyone had ever complained in the past it had done no good. Or maybe they got into trouble for complaining, and they got labeled "the newcomer who is a troublemaker". So everyone was used to her ways and accepted it as a normal procedure. Complaining would thus not bring about good results.

If you as the newcomer complain, you will look like the bad person, plus the charge nurse might feel you were causing trouble. Instead of complaining, just do your own job, don't look at how anyone else is doing his or her work. The only time that a new nurse should risk complaining about another nurse is if his or her behavior prevents the new nurse from doing her own job.

Remember you shouldn't do a job for anyone else. This just causes a lot of trouble, mostly for you. You must just worry about doing your own job and not looking at anyone else's. New people have to do their job to the fullest because every one is watching them. No one is watching the nurse who has been there for years. You may wonder why some nurses get away with murder and you can't get away with anything. Well, you are the new nurse and what the new nurses have to do is totally different from what a nurse who has been there a long time has to do. The difference between them is like night and day. You may think that you are doing someone a favor or getting something done the right way, but it will seem like you are complaining about how things are done. Now it will seem as though the newcomer wants to show the people in the department the right way of doing things. No one likes being told or shown that they have been doing things the wrong way, even if it is true and done nicely. Eventually resentment of that person occurs. So stick to the old familiar procedures even if you think you know a better way.

Instead, try to blend in and not create new procedures for doing things. The procedures have been done a certain way for years. Remember that people are comfortable with what they know. They will not feel comfortable with you if you try to change their long-standing procedures or change their familiar ways. Also, try to work in a group, because there is protection in numbers. This way none of the group members alone will get accused of saying or doing something out of the ordinary. You'd all be there as witnesses and protectors for each other. Be the follower in the group. Let a nurse who has been there for a long time take the leading role. She knows the procedures of the hospital and you will comfortably ease in.

How to Say No

There will be times when you will be put in a situation that you feel you can't handle and you will have to decline for the safety of the patient. There are ways of declining without offending the supervisor or putting your position in jeopardy. You may find yourself assigned to a procedure that you had not performed recently or required to use equipment that may be more complicated than you expected. You may be a floor nurse who is sent to intensive care, labor and delivery or the emergency room. If you voice your concerns to the charge nurse you may be told that other nurses will help you so you will be fine doing it. If you still feel uncomfortable, another voicing of your concerns will be perceived as complaining and unwillingness to help and will likely be brought up in your annual performance review.

So what do you do? If you just say "No" you can be fired unless a contract to the contrary exists. There are ways of making difficult situations like these manageable. First, ask the opinion of your co-workers. Chances are they have been in a similar situation before and know the best way for you to proceed. Or at least they can tell you what they did wrong when trying to solve it. Take the advice of your co-workers and proceed cautiously.

If the senior staff nurse is asking you to do duties you don't feel comfortable with and she is not understanding you concerns, you may want to go talk to the supervisor. Make sure before you do this whether it is a beneficial route to take. You don't want to find out after the fact that the supervisor usually never does anything against the senior staff nurse wishes and now the staff nurse is mad at you for going to the supervisor. If you do go to the supervisor, explain that you are there to help and you want to do a good job but you feel it would be in the best interest of the patients if you were assigned to do a procedure you feel comfortable doing. This is usually your last resort. Do this after you have tried everything else.

Some rules for saying, "No", to achieve best results:
Ask co-workers for advice and help.
Nicely talk to your charge nurse and tell her your concerns, giving alternative duties that you will be willing to do instead
If talking to your charge nurse failed, find out whom the best person to talk to is, maybe the union representative or her supervisor. This should be the last resort.

Laws

The Supreme Court has not always been an ally to nurses. In one case a nurse was fired for insubordination by a hospital when she complained about the working conditions in her department and this was reported to her supervisor. It was stated that employees can be fired for making insubordination statements even if they made other statements that would be constitutionally protected free speech and that the employer used due care that a reasonable manager would use before making an employment decision. This means an employer cannot be held liable for firing someone who they believed made statements unprotected by free speech.

Complaining can get complicated. As a new nurse keep it to a minimum and follow the rules outlined in this chapter and you should succeed in accomplishing productive constructive complaining.

Conclusion

Complaining is part of life. This chapter helped you learn how to use complaining for your best results. There are two forms of complaining, constructive and unconstructive complaining. Constructive complaining is when you know how and to whom to complain to bring about positive results. Unconstructive complaining is done the wrong way to the wrong person at the wrong time thus causing more harm than good.

The steps to constructive complaining outlined in this chapter will help you know how and to whom to complain to get positive results. Do your research; get to know the people and policies of the hospital before you constructively complain. If you complain too often, it will eventually mean nothing. The supervisors hired you to do a job, not to make their job harder, so be cautious when complaining to supervisors. Make sure your complaints are not going to make their job harder.

Doctors /nurse relationships were discussed. Hints on handling criticism, abuse and sexual harassment by doctors were discussed and ideas were given to best deal with these situations. Hints such as trying never to confront a doctor in the presence of a patient and stay silent in certain situations until the crises is over were revealed.

Relationships between nurses should be healthy, congenial, cooperative and friendly. Behavior that will help you accomplish this was given in this chapter by way of a self-evaluation questionnaire. Optimistic and pessimistic attitudes were discussed and how they affect views about complaining. The roles of outside work interests and needs of nurses in order to find balance in life thus keeping complaining in its proper place was stated. How to say, "No" in a diplomatic way was revealed and easy steps given on how to achieve this.

New nurses should be very careful who and what they complain about and they should also keep complaining to a minimum. They are at a disadvantage. Remember that you are the new person so you have to conform to the social rules of the hospital in order to fit in. Don't try to change things, no one likes someone to tell them how things should be done differently. Everyone likes familiar ways, so if you try to change their familiar ways, they will not like it or you. Be optimistic. Be sensitive to others and try to understand others' point of view. Try to find a balance in your life. Balance in work, health, social and leisure activities is essential. Try to blend in, do your own job, and don't try to change a lot at once. You can learn to make complaining work for you.

Notes

1. Jane Schweitzer, RN, M.P.A., *Tears and Rage*, (Adams-Blake Publishing 1993)

2. Janet Kraegel, RN, Mary Kachoyeanos, RN, *Just a Nurse*, (E.P. Dutton 1989)

Chapter 10

The Ten Commandments of Nursing

The Ten Commandments of Nursing
1. Find the right environment for your professional goals
2. Interact cooperatively with physicians
3. Follow policies, procedures and nursing standards
4. Don't alienate your co-workers
5. Don't put your own beliefs ahead of the patient's
6. Don't alienate the patient's family
7. Choose your work friends cautiously
8. Complain Constructively
9. Don't Monopolize Meetings
10. Do extra's for the supervisors

1. Find the right environment for your professional goals

Now that you have examined your goals you have a better understanding of what you want and why. You are aware of which institutions, position and salary levels would be best for you and how to obtain them. Use families, friends, organizations, etc. to find information about the nursing position you are applying for. Get as much information about the position before you go for the interview. Then you will know if it is the right position for you.

Remember that supervisors-especially charge nurses are the most important people in the facility. Not only do they set the whole tone on the floor, they have the power to influence your evaluations, promotions, hiring and firing, shifts, and general acceptance. Supervisors can easily make your life wonderful or miserable. You should try to work under a supervisor who likes you. This is the number one thing you need in order to succeed in easing into any health facility. In fact, it is probably the only thing you need. You can have everything else, but if you don't have a fair supervisor preferably one who like you. You have nothing.

Usually, when you accept your first position you will not have a choice of a charge nurse especially if you request a certain unit or department. Find out as much as you can about the charge nurse, if she seems fair then it will probably be a good idea to take the position. If you hear very negative comments about her you may want to work in another unit with a charge nurse with a fair reputation. If you do find yourself in a hostile atmosphere there is no need to stay there. Move on, nurses are in demand you don't have to stay where you are unhappy. You can probably find a better environment.

The relationship between nurse and charge nurse seems to have an extraordinary effect. It models how all relationships will be. The new nurse has to learn to understand the views of the charge nurse. You have to start to learn the views, needs, and wants of the charge nurse and other supervisory nurses even at your own expense, so that you can achieve harmony in the workplace. If you make the charge nurse's job easier then he/she will like you and want you in their unit.

Find the right facility for you. In addition to the traditional hospital setting, you can work in personal care facilities, offices and clinics of physicians, offices and clinics of health practitioners (chiropractors, optometrist's etc.), home care, kidney dialysis centers, drug treatment clinics, rehabilitation centers, blood banks, schools as well as general industry. Also find the facility that has the closest views on health care as you do. You now have decided which concerns are the most significant to you and know how to choose which facility would be right for you.

You now know how much education you will need for whatever position you decided to take. You also know how much the approximate salary and what your duties would be.

Before you go on any interviews, find out as much about the institution, position and charge nurse as you can. This is where family, friends and networking play an important role. Even if your family or friends can't hire you they can inform you of certain supervisors and their personalities. The most important element in your success as a nurse is whom you work under. So try to work under someone who likes you and who is fair. Find out as much as you can about the charge nurse or nurses you will be working under. By doing this you will have a good prospective of what your job will entail and if you can conform to it. Interview at the facilities that you feel will be the best environment for you.

Remember the nurse supervisors/charge nurses are the most important people to your successful induction into nursing. The first and most important thing to do when trying to ease into any health facility is to find a fair nurse a superior who likes you. Also find the facility and position that best suits your needs and professional goals and you will have a successful induction into the nursing field..(Refer to Chapters 1 and 2)

2. Interact cooperatively with physicians

Physicians are another form of supervisor, they indirectly have control of a lot that can effect your success as a nurse. In order to succeed as a nurse you will have to learn to compromise and get along with the physicians. Your relationship with a physician can vary considerable depending on the personality of the physician. It can run from treating you with respect to being treated like you were a servant. Nurses usually work directly with the attending physicians. You have to do your homework and find out about the personalities of the physicians and the best way to handle them. Your co-workers will be a good source of information for this.

If possible try not to confront a physician, especially in front of a patient. In the cases where you feel it would be beneficial to confront the physician be careful about how and where you do so, otherwise the physician may retaliate on you or the patient. You also have to be careful about not getting in between a patient and the physician. Nurses who are openly assertive can be labeled aggressive. Once the physicians labeled you aggressive there is a chance no one will want to work with you. You lost your credibility. You can continue to be assertive and insist on doing nursing things, but the physicians may challenge every decision you make. So be careful how you go about getting your nursing done. Do it in a way that doesn't irritate the physician.

Even after you have established a good working relationship with physicians, they will probably do things to protect themselves. The bottom line is that doctors are going to protect themselves. They can seem like your friend but in a questionable case of malpractice they look after their own license. Years ago the doctor was considered the captain of the ship and only he would be sued but today they go for the whole team. Nurses beware, don't let your hospital tell you that you will be covered under the hospital's insurance policy. Get your own. Become aware of this and protect yourself, don't be naïve and think the physicians are going to always be fair to you. Most physicians are fair and cooperative but there is a small percent that might not be, so be aware but optimistic. (Refer to Chapters 4)

3. Follow policies, procedures and nursing standards

Any health care facility you work for is a business and you will have to learn to abide by its policies in order to succeed. Sometimes, because of federal regulations certain constraints are placed on the health care facilities that causes ethical problems. In order to cope with the issues in the nursing profession you will have to learn the policies and procedures of the institution where you work. Cost is a big thing in hospitals today. Saving money, finding the cheapest vendors for hospital supplies is an important aspect of this. Also nurses have to sell their preventive services to the institution that are concerned with money. You have to demonstrate saving through prevention. Every department has a nurse standard of care that you will have to abide by.

For instance, most hospitals have only a certain number of Medicare patients that they will accept. They have to keep the number of paying patients at a certain level to make a profit. Turning away Medicare patient might not seem ethical but it is something that is done and a nurse will have to get used to it. Also, the type of hospital that you work for such as a religious verses a public or private may determine the polices that the hospital expects their nurses to follow. (Refer to chapter 3)

You may have a conflict within yourself when you become a nurse on the issues of, "What should I be doing as opposed to what the institutional values are". Sometimes you will find yourself doing what the institution wants you to do as opposed to what you believe you ought to be doing. There may be a difference between your values and the polices and practices of the institution where you work. No one wants to tell you this but this conflict does exist and you will have to learn to deal with it when you become a nurse. If you accept that there will be a conflict no matter where you work, you can then find a place that has the least amount of conflicting issues and work there. Find out about the polices and procedures of the institution before you accept the position. Talk to friends and family who are associated with the institution and can give you insight into the issues.

You must learn to cover your back, whether by documenting or while delivering care. It may sometimes feel like motivation based on fear but lives are in your hands and that can be very scary. Following the rules, regulations and polices of the facility will help you cover your back and ease into nursing. (Refer to Chapter 3)

4. Don't Alienate Your Co-Workers

Your co-workers are your most valued source of information and support. You need them to help you adjust to almost any situation. You want to become one of the group, you don't want to alienate anyone of them. Most people achieve genuine intimacy with only a few people in their lifetime. You are not likely to bond with those significantly different from yourself, but it is crucial that you understand the role they play in your world. The more diversified the staff, the more difficult interaction becomes. A large city public hospital will have the most diversity among the staff. This diversity usually diminishes as the size of the hospital decreases. The smaller hospitals will probably have a more uniform staff while private and religious hospitals will more likely have the most homogeneous staff.

Every department, floor unit or ward has its own personality. Some department's personnel will be more compatible to your personality than others. There are department's that have an all for one, one for all team spirit among the staff. Then there are departments that are not so congenial and may have cliques that divide the staff. You will have to learn to fit into whatever the situation.

There are some basic rules for interacting with your colleagues to ensure cohesive interaction, such as: Don't criticize or outwardly disagree with another nurse in front of a patient, family member, or at a staff meeting. Talk to a nurse privately about a problem. Choose your cliques of nurses and eat lunch with them if possible. Don't do anyone else's job unless you are asked to by a supervisor. Reciprocate any favors that are given to you.

It is essential that you develop an admirable co-working relationship with your colleagues. You are the new person and you will have to learn to fit in not the other way around. Most people are nice and want to help and include the new person. Just use the rules outlined and you will ease into any nursing position. (Refer to Chapters 3, 4,5 and 9)

5. Don't put your own beliefs ahead of the patient's

Your own beliefs will have to come second to the patients. In order to succeed as a nurse you will have to carry out the beliefs and decisions of the patient. The patient's wishes should always come before your own unless it's against the law. You may know what would really help them, but if the patient's doesn't want it, you simply cannot do it. You have to harden up and face the fact that you are not going to help every patient the way you think is best: rather, you are going to help the patient in the best way the patient allows you to.

Both you and the patient will have to conform to the doctors, institution and family wishes. When you care for a patient, realize that you have to abide by their wishes, their families' wishes, their physicians' wishes and the facilities wishes. After you accept this you can more easily care for the patient.

Caring for patients entails more then just physical care. You have to mentally care for them as well. Some patients need more care then others and some will affect you more emotionally then others. Not only are you caring for them physically, you are caring for them emotionally as well.

You may find it hard when a patient does not decide on the best health solution. Your main aim is to encourage the patient to find his own solutions based on information he has been given. You can suggest solutions based on the doctors and medical facility procedures. What needs to be clarified is that the patient makes the decision and you abide by it. Even when the patient is unconscious, you have an obligation to know what their wishes are and carry them out.

Avoid giving the patient a solution yourself. Guide the patient into finding his own comfortable solution. You should only offer a solution when a patient has exhausted all his ideas and found none to be acceptable. Then proceed with caution. Try not to impose your beliefs on the patient but instead listen to their wishes and help them carry them out. The best decision is the one the patients make themselves and it may not coincide with yours (Refer to Chapter 8)

6. Don't alienate the patient's family

It is very important that you form a good relationship with the patient's family. If you alienate them in any way this can cause problems for you as well as the patient. You will have to find the best spot between the families, patient, physician and the hospital. The patient's illness can be in part the product of their family and life. Patients and their illness are better addressed when you have family cooperation.

When the family and home life are positive, these patients will probably heal faster. If the patient comes from an unstable family where he has little support this may effect his healing in a negative way. Although there are exceptions there seems to be a connection between the patient's family and the healing process. Patterns of family visits and connection to the treatment of the patients will mirror your patient's progress.

Sometimes you will get satisfaction from your work just because you didn't get any family complaints. Some nurses feel intimidated by strong families and others like and seek the families out. Either way will work and you will find which works best for you. Nurses and families are on the same side in that they both want to do what is best for the patient. Therefore if you look at families as allies, then you can establish communication.

As a nurse you cannot expect your professional authority to go unquestioned, for sometimes families will question your nursing skills and you will have to be able to defend yourself.

There are many different types of families. There are families who can make a nurse' life miserable for the whole time she takes care of the patient, by constant phone calls and question about the treatment. There are some families who believe by virtue of having to pay the hospital bill that they can expect nurses to serve as the patient's private caregiver. Then there are the families that are most grateful to the nurse for whatever she does.

Despite the difficulty that nurses sometimes feel when confronted by an occasionally intrusive family member it is less worrisome than the habitually absent one. Most nurses want and seek family involvement for their patients. There are many factors that promote or inhibit participation in the patient's care. Unquestionably, some family members' life circumstances, wealth, work, health, or family obligation influence the extent of their involvement and the patterns of involvement.

There are many different types of families you will encounter. Some helpful hints for success when dealing with any type of family are; Check the names and relations to the patient of all involved, be cordial in your greeting, answer all questions about the treatment in an honest but positive way, never give information that only the physician should reveal, try not to take comments personally, listen carefully and let them participate, present the positive and the negative, but start with the positive, be sensitive to the nonverbal, call the attending physician if need arises, and never be negative about the patient's progress.

Most families are cooperative, but there are a few uncooperative families. Don't jeopardize your job for these types of families. Make sure you abide by the guidelines of the physician, your co-workers, and patient and stay within the polices of the institution. (Refer to Chapters 6 and 8)

7. Choose Your Work friends Cautiously

There are friends outside of work, and then there are friends from work. If a person has to choose between a friendship they formed at work and their job itself, nine times out of ten the person will pick the job. People are there to work, not to socialize, especially if they have mortgages, rents, loans, kids in college, etc. Everyone wants to be friendly but when push comes to shove, they want their jobs more.

Nurses look to colleagues to meet their personal needs for social interaction, reassurance, and psychological support. The format and activities that serve each of these purposes differ. Nurses who conceive of nursing as a largely independent activity might rely on peers to meet personal needs superficially, while nurses who recognize the interdependent nature of nursing might seek collaboration closely with colleagues.

Some experienced nurses feel it is their responsibility to assist an incoming nurse who may be experienced or a complete novice, and work with them through the year, to be their friend, to answer questions, and to try to anticipate areas where they might need help. Most of the time these are very nice nurses who really want to help you. On occasion, you may find a nurse who has other reasons for wanting to help you. You have to make sure your relationship stays as informal assistance rather then formal supervision. Unless she is the charge nurse or another type of supervisor.

Nurses who talk about everyone can be dangerous, especially if they are talking to supervisors. Try to find out who goes to the supervisors. A hint, they would be the ones that you see sitting and socializing with the supervisors. First, always be friendly to them. If they really annoy you try to avoid them. Second, if you can't avoid them be involved with them as little as possible. If you don't have a good feeling about them try not to have them learn your problems, never ask them for favors, and never disagree with them. Try to get on their good side without getting involved in their circle. Bide your time until you get the experience and the acceptance of your supervisors.

Please don't get the wrong impression, most nurses are genuinely friendly and nice. Don't isolate yourself from the staff. New nurses are far more likely to achieve success if they find colleagues to help them through the uncertainties and hazards of nursing. Just pick carefully what nurses you have help and how.

Most people achieve genuine intimacy with only a few people in their lifetime. You are unlikely to bond with those totally different from yourself, but it is crucial that you understand the role that they play in your world. The staff of a facility is not usually a band of similar people, but rather a wide range of different strangers that must make a healthy diverse staff. It is a society where people who would not naturally experience intimacy with each other nonetheless learn to share a common territory and common values for the sake of the patients.

The overwhelming majority of nurses maintain close relationships with only a few colleagues, often members of a team or subset of a department. You will probably become friendly with a few of your colleagues and you will need this support and interaction. It will also help you ease into a department. Every department has its own personality. Some department's personnel will be more compatible to your personality than others. There are departments that have an all for one, one for all spirit among the staff. Then there are departments that are not so congenial and they may have cliques that divide the staff.

The first few months you should be on guard and talk to the people you work with as if you were talking to a supervisor. Sometimes when you first get a position, people will befriend you only to gain information. They may want this information for all sorts of reasons. Maybe they want to place you in the social ladder somewhere and they need to find out whom you know and how much clout you have. Or maybe they are worried about their own positions and want to know why you were hired and what credentials you have. Of course, there are some that are just naturally curious and friendly and want to help you. You won't be able to differentiate between any of them for a little while.

Always, and especially when you first get the position, be friendly to but cautious with everyone. After the first year or so it will become evident who your friends will become. A fairly good rule to follow in ensuring an easy initiation into a department is to always make friends with the supervisors the first few years. They are the only ones who can help you to keep your job. You want to get into a department where the charge nurse/nurse relationships are relaxed, close, helpful, trusting and stable.

The other workers will like you just because you are friendly with the supervisor. If the supervisors doesn't like you and you are at risk of losing your job soon, you would be shocked at how fast most of your friends from work will treat you as if you had the plague. They would be afraid to be around you, because they might catch what you have and also lose their job. So make friends with people who can help you first and then think about socializing. It will all fall into place if you are friendly with the supervisors. (Refer back to chapter 2.)

8. Complain Constructively

Constructive complaining is when you know how and to whom to complain to bring about positive results. There may be times when you will be tempted to complain but before you do make sure you have done your research and know the constructive way to complain for positive results. Have a plan and give valued constructive criticism to ensure the best results.

Learn to complain constructively. Complain to the people who can really help. Make sure you complain to the right person in the right way at the right time. Find out the proper protocol for complaining in the facility. Is the best protocol to go straight to the nurse supervisor or to the charge nurse or do you go to the union representative with constructive complaints first? Find the right person to complain to. Find out the relationships people have within the departments. Do your research and find out what ways works best with what person.

If, as a new comer you are displeased at the way things are done, think twice before you voice these opinions. You don't know how they will be received. Most people do not like change and if you are suggesting change they may decide to change you instead. So think carefully before you complain. You have to find out whom to go for help. If you decide to complain you might as well make sure you complain to someone who can help you. Complain only if you feel there is a good chance you will get something improved and not put yourself in a bad situation.

Steps to constructive complaining are, make sure complaining will accomplish good results, complain to the right person, and find out how to complain properly to that person. Use proper department protocols; do research on peoples' relationships before complaining. Inexperienced nurses should be very careful if complaining about other nurses. New nurses should keep complaints to a minimal or nil. Don't complain if it's going to make the supervisors work harder. Don't complain when you are angry and don't constantly complain to co-workers.

If you complain to much about how things are run, as a newcomer it will seem as if you are trying to show everyone the errors of their ways. Now it will seem as though you think you can show them how to do it the right way. Remember that these jobs have been done a certain way for years, and that people are comfortable with what they know. They will not feel comfortable with you if you try to change their comfortable procedures. Instead try to blend in and not make up new ways of doing things. (Refer back to chapter 9)

9. Don't Monopolize Meetings

Meetings can be wonderfully friendly and informative gatherings, or they can be anxiety ridden torture devices in which people are demanding and accusatory. When you go to a meeting, be prepared for anything and everything. Try not to say too much, to be the center of attention, or to be the one to whom they must explain things. You don't want to look too stupid or too smart. Try to find the middle ground. Find out as much as you can about the meeting's agenda before you actually get there.

There are many different types of meetings: staff meetings, family/patient meetings, and patient interviews. Staff meetings are usually part of a large hospital's agenda. They are informative and will help you learn what you need to know to take care of the patients on your floor. Usually the charges nurse or nurse supervisor leads the staff meetings. The task of the leader is very important in maintaining a satisfactory balance. They have most of the power and can make or break a meeting's harmony. Also, always agree with the supervisors, especially at a meeting. Even the nicest supervisors will find it hard to take criticism in front of others. Agree with him at all costs because it will only hurt you if you don't.

The assessment interview with the patient will set the scene for planning appropriate care for the patient. The important things to remember for this type of meeting are where, when, the amount of privacy you will have, and the time allotted. The right time is when the patient feels comfortable talking, the amount of time is related to how the time is used and privacy is what the patient feels safe enough to disclose information in.

There are other types of parent, family health provider meetings.

The physicians will be the lead with most of the family patient meetings. If you are present just keep a low profile and agree with the physician.

Whatever the situations meetings are an important part of nursing. You can make any type of meeting work for you. (Refer to chapter 7)

10. Do extras for the supervisors

The supervisors are the biggest influence in whether or not you can ease into a department or not. Usually, you should do whatever a supervisor reasonably asks you to do. As a newcomer you may think that you have rights, but you really don't have many. If you want a job, you are going to have to impress your supervisors. Maybe an experienced nurse has rights and so they don't have to do everything that a nurse supervisor asks them to do. But you, as a newcomer do not have that privilege. So befriend your supervisors, let them know you are there for them and that you will do whatever they reasonably ask. If they are fair, then they will not take advantage of you. If they are unfair, you will soon find this out as you try to please them. You will soon know whether they are people that you can work for or not. If you find yourself trying to please a supervisor, but nothing you do is ever good enough, then you know that you are working for the wrong person. In this case try to leave as soon as possible.

The nurse supervisor relationship is one in which the supervisor does have some control, power and the upper hand. Many supervisors view themselves as the policy makers of the department and view the nurses as executives whose task it is to make that policy operational. A real affiliation problem can arise when a supervisor holds this view and the nurse doesn't.

Nurses are dependent on their supervisors for keeping their position, for references, and for various favors such as duty assignments. Ignoring the importance of this relationship can adversely affect a nurse's success.

The supervisors are swamped with work, and if they have people on their staffs who are willing to do extra jobs, they will know you are on their side and they will want you in their department, if they are fair, that is. Remember, the only one who can help you keep your job when you first get into a department, is you and your supervisor. So befriend him or her, try to help the supervisor when you can. Get on his or her team, and if he or she is fair, you will find that you will have successfully eased into a facility. (Refer back to chapter 2.)

Conclusion

The nursing profession is one of the most rewarding careers you can choose. You can make a difference in many peoples lives while touching the future and leaving your imprint on the world. It can be an extremely heroic or it can be a trivial kind of job. What, a nurse does ranges from the most mundane, like helping patients go to the bathroom to the most sublime like helping the patient find peace and healing. It is a perplexing profession filled with contradictions and predictions. Sometimes when you try your very best it isn't going to be good enough. You have the stress of holding a patient's life in your hands while trying to juggle the rules and regulation that you must follow. It can be both an extremely frustrating and rewarding career. But one important contact with a patient, one good deed or good care can justify it all. Go out and succeed in the nursing profession. You are very needed.

Author's Biography

Marianne Pilgrim Calabrese earned her Masters Degree in Reading from Adelphi University. Her Bachelor degree from Queens College is in Elementary Education and Psychology. She is a published author and renowned artist. She has extensive classroom reading experience and has conducted workshops for the New York City Board of Education in Curriculum and Testing. She is currently serving on the Executive Board of Directors of the Nassau Reading Council, and has also received, "The Presidents' Club Award" from the International Reading Association for her work.

To research her new book, Marianne spent many hours studying nursing journals and related books. She interviewed numerous nurses and doctors and spent months volunteering at different types of medical institutions.

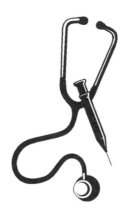